GUT HEALTH, MICROBIOME & METABOLISM RESET FOR
WOMEN OVER 50

Reclaim your vitality with an inner health reset—reduce cortisol, improve digestion, boost brain power, and support natural weight loss in your golden years

ED NEELSEN

Author's Note on Case Studies & Names

The personal stories, case studies, and experiences shared in this book are drawn from real-life situations.

To protect the privacy of individuals, some names and identifying details have been changed. Any resemblance to actual persons, living or dead, is purely coincidental.

These narratives are intended to illustrate the emotional and practical aspects of healing, not to diagnose or prescribe.

Contents

Introduction

Have you ever noticed how your body speaks to you differently now than it did just a few years ago? Maybe the foods you used to enjoy now leave you feeling uneasy, suddenly feeling bloated, tired or just "off" Your energy seems to fade without warning and no matter how much rest you get, you still feel drained. These changes can feel confusing—but you're not alone and you're not imagining things.

Something powerful is happening inside you. Within your body lies an extraordinary universe – your gut microbiome. This ecosystem of trillions of bacteria plays a bigger role in your life than you may realize. It works tirelessly to support your health, fuels your immune system, and even your emotions. For women over 50, this delicate ecosystem faces unique challenges that can affect everything from digestion to brain function, energy levels, to emotional wellbeing.

This book is your invitation to reconnect—with your body, your health, and your vitality. Drawing from both ancient wisdom and modern science, we'll discover how stress affects digestion, why certain foods may be silently disrupting your system, and most importantly, how to reset your gut health for optimal vitality in your golden years. You'll find practical and accessible solutions that fit your lifestyle and budget, helping you navigate this important stage of life with confidence and ease.

Whether you're dealing with digestive issues, struggling with low energy levels, or simply seeking to understand your body better, this book offers a roadmap to renewal. Through real-life stories of women who have walked this same road and transformed their health by understanding their gut, you'll find hope, inspiration, and practical guidance for your own journey.

Your body isn't your enemy – it's your most faithful ally. When you learn to listen to its wisdom and provide the support it needs, remarkable healing becomes possible. No matter where you are on your health journey, it's never too late to reset, rebuild, and reclaim your vitality from the inside out.

You won't find perfection or pressure here. Instead, you'll find encouragement, clarity, and a gentle roadmap that meets you where you are.

So take a deep breath, open your mind to new possibilities, and prepare to embark on a journey of discovery and renewal. Your healing journey begins here, one mindful step at a time. Together, we'll unlock the secrets of your gut health and help you thrive in ways you never thought possible after 50.

Reflection Prompt

What changes have I noticed in my body over the years? How might these be signals asking for deeper care or attention?

CHAPTER 1
Understanding Your Inner Universe — Reset Your Mind, Reset the Aging Myth

"I embrace the wisdom of my changing body and trust in its natural ability to heal and thrive."

Your Inner Universe: Where Renewal Begins

Inside each of us lies a vibrant ecosystem — more diverse than a rainforest and more influential than we once imagined — our *gut microbiome*. As we journey into our golden years, this inner world evolves and impacts everything from energy to emotional wellbeing.

Every morning, billions of microscopic allies awaken within your gut, quietly influencing your digestion, mood, immunity, and even mental clarity. Yet, many women over 50 overlook the signals this inner ecosystem sends, often mistaking natural transitions of aging for signs of irreversible decline.

What's often missed is this powerful truth: your gut responds not only to what you eat, but also to how you think and feel. Recent studies, including those published in *Nature* and *Science*, highlight the gut's profound role in everything from immune strength to emotional balance.

As we move through this vibrant stage of life, learning to care for our gut isn't just important—it's essential. With the right knowledge and support, you can nurture this inner world and feel more energized, balanced, and resilient than ever before.

The delicate connection between your gut and overall health takes on new significance after fifty. Just as Sarah, a 63-year-old retired teacher, who once believed that bloating, fatigue, and digestive discomfort were just part of getting older. But everything changed when she began to question those assumptions.

By tuning into her body and making mindful changes, Sarah discovered that vibrant health was still within reach. Her journey—from silently enduring symptoms to reclaiming her energy and well-being—shows just how powerful it can be to understand and support the inner workings of our gut.

Your gut isn't merely a processing centre for food – it's a complex communication hub that influences your immune system, emotional state, and even your thought patterns. Like a carefully tended garden, your microbiome responds to your daily choices, thoughts, and emotions. When you honor this internal wisdom, remarkable healing becomes possible.

Many women over fifty have been conditioned to view physical changes as a decline rather than a transition. Yet research published in reputable journals consistently shows that your body maintains an incredible capacity for renewal at any age. Your digestive system isn't failing you – it's trying to communicate with you in ways that can lead to profound healing and regeneration.

Through Sarah's inspiring journey, we witness how challenging limiting beliefs about aging can create tangible improvements in physical health. When she learned to recognize the connection between her stress patterns and digestive symptoms, particularly before family gatherings, she discovered a profound truth: our gut health is intimately connected to our emotional well-being.

Take a moment now to place your hand on your belly. Feel the warmth, the life force flowing beneath your palm. This is your center of vitality – your second brain – and it's ready to guide you toward greater health and wellbeing. As we explore the intricate connection between your thoughts, your gut, and your overall health, remember this affirmation: 'My body holds deep wisdom, and I choose to listen with compassion and curiosity.'

In the pages that follow, we'll delve deeper into understanding your microbiome, exploring the gut-brain connection, and discovering practical ways to support your digestive health. Whether you're experiencing occasional discomfort or seeking to enhance your overall wellbeing, this chapter will provide you with evidence-based knowledge and practical tools to begin your own journey of transformation.

Remember, this path is uniquely yours. While the principles of gut health we'll explore are universal, how you apply them will be deeply personal. Let's begin this exploration with open hearts and curious minds, ready to discover the remarkable potential that lies within your inner universe – a potential that science increasingly shows remains vibrant and accessible at any age.

Breaking Free from Aging Myths: Rewriting Your Health Story with Understanding Natural Changes After 50

Let's take a closer look at some eye-opening truths about the body after 50—truths grounded in recent scientific discoveries and a deeper understanding of the aging process. For example, research published in the journal *Promotion of Healthy Aging* highlights the body's remarkable ability to adapt, even in our later years. The study shows that certain dietary phytochemicals—natural compounds found in plants—can significantly support gut health and promote graceful aging. This challenges the outdated belief that physical decline is unavoidable. In reality, with the right choices, our bodies are far more resilient than we've been led to believe.

Research now confirms what ancient wisdom always hinted at: the gut is your second brain — a dynamic hub that responds not just to food but to thoughts, stress, and beliefs. When nurtured with care, it holds the key to remarkable renewal, even later in life.

Challenging the Aging Myth

🌼 Claire's Story 🌼

Claire, a 64-year-old artist, once believed digestive issues were her new normal. "I assumed the bloating and fatigue were just part of turning the page past 50," she shared. Like many women, she had accepted this discomfort without question — until she began to question the very story she'd been told about aging.

As Claire learned to gently adjust her meals and manage stress, her symptoms eased. What changed most, however, was her mindset. "The biggest shift," she said, "was learning to work with my body, not against it." She began viewing her body not as something breaking down but as something asking for new care.

Resetting Your Beliefs: What the Science Says

Let's unpack three common aging myths:

- **Myth**: Digestive decline is inevitable after 50
- **Truth**: Research shows gut health can improve at any age with the right foods, rest, and emotional support.

- **Myth**: A sluggish metabolism is permanent
- **Truth**: Metabolic shifts occur, but your *microbiome and hormones* can be rebalanced through movement and nutrition.

- **Myth**: It's too late to change
- **Truth**: The microbiome can diversify and heal within days of simple changes.

Instead of seeing these changes as losses, think of them as invitations to shift how you care for yourself. Aging isn't decline — it's evolution.

The aging process brings natural transitions in how our bodies function. Research published in *'The Impact of the Gut Microbiome on Aging'* highlights how our digestive system adapts over time. Rather than viewing these changes as limitations, we can see them as opportunities to evolve our self-care practices.

Recent studies in psychoneuroimmunology—how our thoughts and emotions affect our immune system and overall health—show a strong link between our thoughts about aging and how our body responds. When we let go of limiting beliefs about what's possible for our health, we open the door to healing and renewed vitality."

This journey isn't about denying the natural changes that come with age—it's about understanding them and responding with informed, compassionate care. Your body isn't breaking down or turning against you. In fact, it's inviting you to listen more closely, to recognize what it needs in this new chapter of life.

As you read on, hold onto this powerful truth: aging brings wisdom, and your body carries an incredible ability to heal, adapt, and renew—no matter your age.

In the sections ahead, we'll dive into practical, science-backed strategies to support your gut health while honoring the unique rhythm of your body and lifestyle.

The Gut-Brain Highway:
How Digestive Health Influences Mood and Cognition

Research shows a fascinating link between our digestive system and brain function, especially as we age. The gut-brain axis is a complex network that significantly impacts our thinking and emotional health.

This connection is not just simple; it's a busy route of communication with neurotransmitters, hormones, and immune cells. Research in 'The gut-brain axis: interactions between enteric microbiota, central and enteric nervous systems' shows how this network affects memory, focus, and emotional resilience.

The growing science around the diet-gut-brain connection provides a strong basis for understanding healthy aging. By eating the right foods, we can create a gut environment that produces helpful compounds for both physical and mental health.

While more research is needed to fully explore these relationships and create targeted interventions, current evidence highlights a diet rich in diverse plant foods as essential for healthy aging. By nurturing our gut microbiome, we also support our brains and bodies, which may lead to a longer, more fulfilling life.

As this field develops, we can look forward to more personalized strategies that consider our unique microbiome, genetics, and health status. In the meantime, a varied, plant-rich diet is our best approach for enhancing the important link between our diet, gut, and brain as we age.

🌷 Linda's Awakening 🌷

Linda, a 65-year-old retired librarian, struggled with mood swings and mental fog. "It felt like my brain wasn't mine anymore," she said. But as she learned about the gut-brain connection, she began to understand the missing piece.

The gut produces over 90% of your body's serotonin — the feel-good hormone — and sends messages to your brain through neurotransmitters, immune signals, and even electrical impulses. A troubled gut clouds the mind, while a nourished gut sharpens it.

Linda created a simple ritual: deep breathing, soft music, and tea before breakfast. "Within weeks," she said, "I felt clearer — like I was waking up mentally for the first time in years."

Linda's transformation began when she started implementing these simple practices. She created a peaceful morning routine that included gentle stretching and a quiet breakfast, free from her usual news feed. 'Within weeks,' she shared, 'I noticed my thinking becoming clearer and my moods more stable.'

Sharing meals with others in a relaxed environment can enhance both digestion and emotional wellbeing. Consider organizing regular gatherings with friends who support your wellness journey.

As we age, this gut-brain connection becomes even more crucial. The good news is that simple, daily practices can strengthen this vital highway, supporting both digestive health and cognitive function.

Linda's story reminds us that it's never too late to enhance this connection. Six months after implementing these changes, she reported not just improved digestion but also enhanced mental clarity and emotional stability. 'I feel more like myself again,' she shared. 'It's as if clearing my gut cleared my mind too.'

Your Microbiome Garden

🌹 Rose's Renewal 🌹

Imagine your gut as a vibrant, living garden— teeming with life and possibility. Like any garden, this internal ecosystem requires mindful tending and care to flourish.

Every food you eat, every habit you practice, and even the thoughts you entertain become part of its soil, shaping its health. Rose, 67, had recurring digestive issues and frequent infections. "I didn't realize my inner garden needed more than just avoiding bad foods — it needed nurturing," she reflected.

When Rose began introducing *fiber-rich vegetables*, fermented foods, and simple, mindful routines into her life, the change was evident. Not only did her digestion improve, she also felt emotionally steadier and more resilient. "I stopped reacting to everything — physically and emotionally," she said. "It felt like balance returned to my body."

Understanding Your Inner Garden

- Your microbiome contains trillions of beneficial bacteria
- These microscopic allies help digest food, produce vitamins, and support immunity
- A diverse microbiome supports both physical and emotional health

The health of your microbiome influences:

- Immune system function
- Nutrient absorption
- Hormone balance
- Emotional wellbeing
- Energy levels

Closing Practice

Place one hand on your belly, one on your heart. Take three deep breaths, counting to four. Feel the air filling your stomach and rising. Slowly breathe out, counting six and feel the belly muscle tucked in with the last bit of air going out. Practice this only with three breaths for a week. Once you master the breathing technique, you can consciously do it at any time to ease the pressure, fatigue or stress. Know that with every mindful choice, you're tending the garden of your wellbeing — one step, one breath, one meal at a time.

Mindset Reset: Journal Prompts

- What beliefs about aging am I ready to release?
- How might my life feel if I treated change as wisdom instead of warning?
- What signals has my body been trying to send me?
- What part of my health story am I ready to rewrite?
- How does my gut feel when I slow down and tune in?

As you continue this journey of gut renewal and graceful aging, take a moment to reflect on how your body speaks to you through food, feelings, and everyday rhythms. Your gut is not just a digestive system—it's a second brain, a wise partner guiding your energy, clarity, and emotional balance. By tuning into what nourishes you—physically and emotionally—you begin to rewrite the parts of your health story that no longer serve you.

Remember, your microbiome is flexible and responsive at any age and aging itself can be a powerful breakthrough rather than a slow breakdown. Start small: keep a gentle food-and-mood journal, enjoy one mindful meal each day, and build rituals that relax your mind and body. Most importantly, speak kindly to yourself—your body is always listening, always adapting, always striving to support your best self.

Next Chapter Preview: Listening to Your Body's Wisdom

Your body is always speaking—sometimes in whispers, sometimes with urgency. In the next chapter, you'll learn how to recognize early signs of gut imbalance and understand the deep connection between your digestion, emotions, and overall well-being. With real-life stories, gentle natural remedies, and practical journaling tools, you'll discover how to tune in, respond with care, and support your gut through every season of life. Aging isn't a breakdown—it's a breakthrough, and your body holds the wisdom to guide the way.

CHAPTER 2
Listening to Your Body's Wisdom:
Signs of Gut Imbalance and Natural Solutions

*"I listen to my body's wisdom
and trust its gentle guidance toward healing."*

Your Body Speaks – Are You Listening?

Our bodies often whisper before they ever raise their voice. But for many women over 50, life's demands can be so consuming that those early signals go unnoticed. Subtle signs of gut imbalance—like occasional bloating, fatigue, or changes in mood—are easy to brush off.

Yet, when left unaddressed, these small whispers can grow into persistent discomfort or chronic health challenges. Much like learning a new language, developing a relationship with your body's cues requires time, curiosity, and a soft willingness to pay attention. The *Journal of Nutrition* and *Biology* affirm that our gut communicates with our brain and immune system in real time — a dialogue that becomes especially vital as we age and our hormones shift.

This fascinating gut-brain connection becomes even more crucial for women over 50, as hormonal changes can amplify the impact of digestive wellness on overall health. Studies published in the Journal of Nutrition have demonstrated that women in their golden years who maintain strong gut health often experience better emotional resilience and clearer cognitive function.

🌷 Margaret's Turning Point: Listening to Her Body 🌷

Take Margaret, 58, who initially dismissed bloating, irritability, and fatigue as "just aging". But, by journaling her meals, stress levels, and symptoms, she began to notice consistent patterns.

By learning to tune into these subtle messages, Margaret discovered that her body wasn't failing her—it was actually trying to guide her toward better choices. She began incorporating gentle herbs like chamomile and peppermint before meals, practiced mindful eating, and made small but significant changes to her diet timing. Six months later, Margaret reported not only improved digestion but also a renewed sense of connection with her body's wisdom. 'I've stopped fighting against my body,' she shared, 'and started listening to what it's been trying to tell me all along.'

"Now I listen to my body like I would a friend."

As we explore the various signs of gut imbalance and natural solutions in this chapter, remember that this journey isn't about achieving perfection. It's about developing a deeper, more compassionate relationship with your body. Your gut's whispers are not inconveniences to be ignored but rather wise messages guiding you toward better health.

Understanding Your Body's Warning Signs: Symptoms of Gut Imbalance

Your body is always communicating—sometimes in ways we don't immediately recognize. According to the journal *Biology*, our digestive system sends out a complex network of signals, each one carrying important messages about our internal balance. When decoded properly, these symptoms can help guide us toward better gut health.

What's important to understand is that gut imbalance doesn't just affect digestion. Because your microbiome is deeply connected to your immune, neurological, and hormonal systems, symptoms often show up in clusters—such as fatigue, skin issues, mood swings, or frequent illness—rather than as one obvious problem. Learning to recognize these patterns is a powerful step toward healing and long-term wellness. Here are some common ones:

- **Digestive Discomfort**: Bloating, gas, constipation, or diarrhea
- **Fatigue**: Especially after meals or in the early afternoon
- **Mood Shifts**: Irritability, anxiety, or low mood tied to food or stress
- **Skin Changes**: Breakouts, rashes, or inflammation
- **Sleep Issues**: Difficulty falling or staying asleep
- **Food Sensitivities**: New discomfort from familiar foods
- **Weight Fluctuations**: Despite stable habits

These symptoms often appear in patterns rather than isolated incidents. Think of them as pieces of a puzzle that, when viewed together, create a clearer picture of your gut health. For instance, you might notice that bloating occurs more frequently after certain meals or that fatigue sets in during particular times of the day.

Try This
- Track your meals, symptoms, and mood for 1–2 weeks
- Reflect on what makes you feel most energized, clear, or sluggish
- Practice a daily body scan — pause, breathe, and tune into how your digestive system feels

The Emotional Connection:
How Mood Changes Signal Gut Health

Our gut and brain are deeply connected through the gut-brain axis — a two-way communication system involving hormones, neurotransmitters, and even immune cells. Up to 95% of serotonin, the "happiness hormone", is produced in the gut. No wonder stress and anxiety disrupt digestion— and poor digestion clouds our emotional wellbeing.

🌸 Janet's Sunday Realisation 🌸

At 64, Janet noticed that her digestive discomfort always spiked on Sunday evenings, just before a stressful workweek. Instead of adding medications, she began journaling emotions, meditating at night, and practicing calm eating rituals. Within weeks, her gut began to settle. "It wasn't just food," she said. "It was fear I hadn't processed."

Common Gut-Emotion Links

- Anxiety → nausea or urgency
- Stress → reflux or indigestion
- Depression → constipation or fatigue
- Joy → smooth digestion and appetite

Remember that emotions aren't something to control or eliminate—they're valuable messengers providing insight into our overall wellbeing. When we learn to listen to and honor our emotional experiences, we often find that improvements in our digestive health naturally follow.

The key is developing awareness without judgment. If you notice anxiety affecting your digestion, respond with gentle understanding rather than criticism. This compassionate approach allows both your nervous and digestive systems to find greater balance.

Recent studies in neurogastroenterology have shown that practicing emotional awareness can actually strengthen the positive communication between our gut and brain, leading to improved digestive function and emotional resilience. This research supports what many traditional healing systems have long understood - that emotional and physical wellbeing are deeply interconnected.

By honoring both our emotional and physical experiences, we create an environment where true healing can flourish. The path to digestive wellness includes making space for all of our emotions - the comfortable and uncomfortable ones alike. As we learn to listen to both our gut and our heart, we discover a deeper wisdom that guides us toward true health.

Gentle, Natural Solutions to Restore Balance

Healing doesn't mean fixing something broken. It means supporting a body that is constantly trying to restore balance. Recent research published in *Science Direct* emphasizes that gentle, natural approaches to gut healing can be highly effective, particularly for women over 50.

The key is working with your body's innate healing capabilities rather than against them. Drawing from both traditional wisdom and modern scientific understanding, let's explore evidence-based solutions that support digestive wellness.

Four Pillars of Natural Gut Healing:

- **Support Beneficial Bacteria** – Polyphenol-rich foods (berries, olive oil, green tea), prebiotics, and fermented foods

- **Reduce Inflammation** – Use turmeric, ginger, omega-3s, and calming rituals
- **Strengthen Gut Barrier** – Bone broth, L-glutamine, zinc, fermented foods
- **Promote Regular Elimination** – Warm water, fiber, gentle movement, herbs

🌷 Clara's Simple Changes 🌷

Clara, 65, struggled with persistent gut discomfort. Instead of overhauling everything, she started small: drinking lemon water in the morning, sipping ginger tea at night, practicing slow eating, and taking evening walks. "Natural solutions," she shared, "helped me trust my body again."

Studies have shown that simple dietary modifications can significantly impact gut health. Research in the journal *'Biology'* highlights the importance of polyphenol-rich foods in promoting beneficial gut bacteria.

Beyond food choices, research demonstrates the effectiveness of gentle herbs in supporting digestive health:

- Peppermint for digestive comfort
- Chamomile for gut-brain calming
- Ginger for motility support
- Turmeric for inflammation reduction
- Marshmallow root for mucosal support

Practical implementation is the key. Start by incorporating one new supportive practice each week.

Movement is one of the most overlooked yet powerful tools in natural gut healing. Research published in the *Journal of Gastroenterology* confirms that even gentle physical activity can enhance gut motility—the wave-like motion that moves food through the digestive tract—and help reduce inflammation. Practices such as morning stretching, slow post-meal walks, gentle yoga, tai chi, or deep breathing exercises not only support digestion but also calm the nervous system, ease stress, and bring the body into a more balanced state.

These simple movements invite your gut to function more smoothly while restoring a sense of connection between body, breath, and mind. In healing, it's often the softest steps that make the biggest difference. The timing of our meals can also significantly impact gut health. Studies on circadian rhythms and digestion suggest that allowing adequate space between meals supports optimal digestive function.

Emerging research on circadian biology shows that the timing of our meals is just as crucial as their content. Leaving a 3-to-4-hour gap between meals gives your gut sufficient time to complete vital processes such as motility and microbial cleanup. This natural pause supports smoother digestion, reduces inflammation, and enhances nutrient absorption. It's not about restriction; it's about giving your body space to do what it was designed to do. Honoring these internal rhythms strengthens the gut and promotes long-term vitality. Healing your gut doesn't have to mean sweeping lifestyle overhauls. In fact, small, steady changes often lead to the most lasting results. Studies show that for women over 50, gentle, consistent shifts are often more effective than intense interventions.

Another key piece of the healing puzzle is stress management. Science continues to confirm the powerful link between emotional well-being and gut health—when we reduce stress, we also reduce digestive distress. Managing stress isn't a luxury—it's a necessity for true, lasting gut healing.

Recent studies have shown that chronic stress can disrupt the delicate balance of the gut microbiome, weaken the gut lining, and trigger inflammation. By reducing stress, we allow the digestive system to function more efficiently and repair itself more naturally. Practices like mindful breathing, journaling, time in nature, and quiet moments of reflection can ease the nervous system, creating a calm inner environment where the gut can heal. In many cases, it's not just what we eat—but how we feel—that shapes our digestive health. Managing stress isn't a luxury—it's a form of nourishment.

Sleep quality also significantly impacts gut health. Research shows that quality sleep supports the body's natural healing processes.

Sleep and stress are deeply intertwined with gut health, forming a quiet foundation for the body's healing process. When stress levels rise, digestion often slows or becomes erratic, while poor sleep weakens the gut barrier and disrupts the microbial balance. Studies now show that chronic stress and sleep deprivation can significantly impair digestion, increase inflammation, and even alter the gut-brain connection.

On the flip side, gentle stress-reducing practices—like evening walks, meditation, or calming herbal teas—paired with consistent sleep routines help regulate cortisol, repair the gut lining, and restore balance to the microbiome. Prioritizing rest and emotional calm isn't just self-care—it's a healing strategy. When your nervous system feels safe, your gut feels safe too.

Consider these gentle sleep-supporting practices:

- Creating a calm bedtime routine
- Using relaxing herbs like chamomile
- Keeping regular sleep/wake times
- Reducing evening screen time

- Creating a peaceful sleep environment

The healing is not about perfection but about progress. Listen to your body's responses and adjust accordingly. What works for one person may not work for another, and that's perfectly normal. The key is finding gentle approaches that resonate with your body and lifestyle.

As you implement these natural solutions, pay attention to how your body responds. Keep a simple journal noting any changes in your digestive comfort, energy levels, and overall wellbeing. This awareness helps you identify which practices provide the most benefit for your unique situation.

Integration: Your Body's Wisdom Is Always Speaking

Throughout our lives, our bodies have been whispering truths—subtle signs, quiet nudges, gentle warnings—but in our youth, vibrant and full of drive, we often raced past them. We were multitasking, chasing goals, looking outward for meaning, with no time to truly listen to the inner child within.

But after 50, those whispers grow louder. They begin to pinch, urging us to wake up from the dream state of doing and return to the wisdom of simply being. The signs are everywhere if we're observant: hair that once felt thick and strong may now feel soft, thin, or brittle—but we blame the shampoo or reach for a new color treatment. Wrinkles emerge gently on the face, but we rush to smooth them with creams instead of asking what stress or imbalance caused them.

Age spots bloom on the skin like tiny messages, but we mask them with makeup. Sagging around the belly or chest isn't just gravity—it's a call to nourish, not neglect. Aching joints in the hips, knees, and ankles are not mere signs of aging but indicators that our foundation needs support, not just supplements. Even brittle nails with lines etched across them speak of internal deficiencies we've long ignored beneath layers of polish.

These are not failures of age—they are reflections of our long-time disconnection. For decades, we fed the brain—our thinking mind—with constant input, pushing productivity, logic, and planning. But we neglected its quiet twin: the gut, our second brain, deeply wired into our nervous system, mood, memory, and immunity. As we cross into our second spring of life, the gut begins to rise, demanding attention. This is not a decline—it's an invitation. A sacred reminder to turn inward and begin a new partnership with our body—one rooted not in fixing but in listening.

Many visible signs of aging are not just due to "getting older" but are strongly linked to deeper imbalances in the gut and its cascading effects on nutrient absorption, inflammation, hormone regulation, and cellular renewal. Below is a detailed, reader-friendly explanation of each symptom, showing how the gut plays a pivotal role in each one:

Hair Thinning and Brittleness

Hair health is directly tied to the nutrients we absorb—particularly protein, iron, B-vitamins (especially Biotin), zinc, and omega-3 fatty acids. When the gut is imbalanced, inflamed, or overloaded with toxins, its ability to absorb these nutrients is compromised. Dysbiosis (an imbalance of gut bacteria) can also trigger chronic inflammation that disrupts the hair growth cycle. Over time, hair may become thinner, softer, or brittle—not just from external products but from internal nutrient loss and hormonal shifts tied to poor gut function.

Wrinkles and Fine Lines

Skin elasticity depends heavily on collagen and hydration, both of which are influenced by gut health. Collagen synthesis requires amino acids and vitamins, such as C and E, which rely on proper digestion and absorption. When the gut is not functioning well, free radicals and inflammatory markers rise, breaking down skin collagen and accelerating wrinkle formation. It's not just the passage of time; it's often the quiet degradation from within.

Age Spots and Pigmentation

What we call "age spots" are often a sign of oxidative stress. A leaky gut can allow toxins and undigested food particles to enter the bloodstream, increasing systemic inflammation and oxidative damage. The liver, which works closely with the gut, may also become sluggish, leading to a buildup of toxins that manifest through the skin. These spots aren't just age—they're signs that the detox pathways, including the gut-liver axis, need support.

Skin Softness and Sagging Texture

The skin's tone and firmness depend on structural proteins like collagen and elastin and on adequate hydration. Chronic low-grade inflammation from an imbalanced gut microbiome depletes these resources over time. Estrogen also plays a role in skin firmness, and the gut plays a key role in hormone recycling through the estrobolome, a subset of gut bacteria that metabolizes estrogen. If the gut is unhealthy, hormone imbalances further affect skin texture.

Nail Ridges and Brittleness

Nails are often early indicators of nutrient deficiencies, especially in protein, zinc, magnesium, and biotin—all nutrients absorbed via a healthy gut. Ridges, lines, brittleness, or peeling nails can suggest malabsorption or chronic stress, both of which are often gut-related. Gut inflammation or dysbiosis may also impair the body's ability to utilize nutrients, even if the diet is adequate.

Hip, Knee, and Ankle Weakness or Pain

While joint pain and reduced mobility are commonly chalked up to aging, chronic gut inflammation is often an overlooked contributor. When the gut is out of balance, it can spark widespread inflammation that affects joints and connective tissue—especially in weight-bearing areas like the hips, knees, and ankles. A compromised gut lining (often referred to as "leaky gut") may allow unwanted particles to enter the bloodstream. These particles can trigger immune reactions that mimic autoimmune responses, leading to joint stiffness or pain. On top of that, poor nutrient absorption—another consequence of gut imbalance—means your body may not be getting enough calcium, magnesium, vitamin D, and K2, all of which are essential for maintaining strong bones and flexible joints.

This physical change is often linked to loss of muscle tone, fat redistribution, and weakened connective tissues—all influenced by hormonal changes, which are tightly linked to gut health. The gut helps regulate estrogen and cortisol. Chronic stress, poor gut health, and toxin accumulation lead to increased belly fat (especially visceral fat) and weakened structural support. Sluggish digestion and constipation may also cause abdominal bloating, contributing to the appearance of sagging.

As we age, visible signs such as thinning hair, wrinkles, sagging skin, joint discomfort, and brittle nails are not just cosmetic or inevitable—they are messages from the body signaling internal imbalances, especially in the gut. For years, we may have overlooked these signs while busy with life, relying on external fixes. However, many of these changes stem from poor nutrient absorption, inflammation, and hormonal shifts—all closely linked to gut health. The gut, often called our "second brain," plays a crucial role in maintaining vitality, strength, and resilience. After 50, it's time to tune in, not cover up. Healing begins when we start listening to these signals and treating them as invitations to care for the body from within.

Key Lessons Recap

- Your body communicates early and often
- Gut imbalance shows up in physical, mental, and emotional ways
- Mood, sleep, and digestion are all interconnected
- Gentle habits create sustainable healing
- Awareness is the first step to transformation

Closing Reflection

- What's one symptom you now recognize as a message, not a malfunction?
- What's one practice you're excited to begin this week?
- How would it feel to trust your body fully and without judgment?

Remember, this journey isn't about achieving perfect health - it's about developing a deeper, more compassionate relationship with your body. Scientific evidence shows that when we listen to and honor our body's signals, we create an environment where true healing can flourish.

As you move into the next chapter, carry forward this enhanced awareness of your body's wisdom. Trust that each symptom, each emotion, and each challenge carries valuable information about what your body needs to thrive. Your body speaks a unique language - one that becomes clearer and more meaningful as you practice listening with patience and compassion.

Take a moment now to appreciate how far you've come in understanding your body's signals. This growing awareness is the foundation for all the healing practices we'll explore in the chapters ahead. Remember, your body's wisdom is always available to guide you - sometimes speaking in whispers, sometimes in clearer tones, but always leading you toward better health.

Trust in this journey of discovery. Your body's wisdom, combined with gentle, consistent care, creates the perfect foundation for vibrant health in your golden years.

Next Chapter Preview: Food, Medicine & Mindful Choices

In the next chapter, we'll explore how to bring awareness into what you eat and how you nourish your body — not just with food but with thoughts, routines, and medications. You'll learn how to decode your cravings, choose gut-friendly foods, and avoid the silent inflammation triggers that can derail your progress.

But for now, take a slow breath. Place your hand on your belly. Feel the quiet intelligence within. This is your second brain — wise, intuitive, and always on your side.

Journal Prompt

What recurring signals might your body be using to ask for change? What have you ignored or explained away as "normal" aging?

CHAPTER 3

The Mindful Reset – Transforming Your Relationship with Food, Aging, and Medicine

"My body knows how to heal, and I trust in its wisdom while embracing the support of modern medicine."

Your Healing Starts with Awareness

In a world of endless health advice, managing medication schedules, and changing diets, it's easy to feel overwhelmed — like you're navigating a maze with no clear map. But within you lies something far more powerful than any external prescription: your own body's wisdom. Yet within you lies an innate wisdom about what your body truly needs – a wisdom that emerges when you learn to pause, breathe, and listen to the subtle signals your digestive system sends.

Recent research, including studies published in *The Journal of Clinical Investigation*, shows that our mindset about healing directly affects our body's responses to both food and medicine. This is especially true for women over 50, who experience hormonal shifts and microbiome changes that require more in-depth attention and care.

🌸 Eleanor's Transformative Journey 🌸

Eleanor, a 65-year-old retired nurse whose story beautifully illustrates this transformative journey. Despite her extensive medical background, she found herself caught between conventional wisdom and her body's natural intelligence, struggling with persistent digestive issues and medication side effects. Her breakthrough came not from adding more treatments but from creating space to truly listen to her body's wisdom.

Eleanor, once felt torn between her extensive medical knowledge and her body's quiet cries for help. Years of prescribed treatments and dietary changes had dulled her ability to listen inward. Her turning point didn't come from adding more pills—it came from pausing, listening, and applying both science and intuition. "I began to treat myself like a partner in healing, not just a patient," she shared. "That's when things began to shift."

Mindfulness isn't an alternative to medicine—it's a bridge between what the body knows and what medicine can offer.

The transition into our golden years often brings unique challenges in managing both our health and our healthcare. We may find ourselves navigating multiple medications, adapting to changing dietary needs or questioning long-held beliefs about aging and wellness. Yet within these challenges lies an opportunity for profound transformation—a chance to develop a more mindful, integrated approach to our wellbeing, supported by emerging research on the gut-brain axis and its role in healthy aging.

This chapter helps you build that bridge: through mindful eating, emotional reflection, and a new relationship with medicine grounded in trust, not fear.

Furthermore, it will guide you through evidence-based strategies for developing a more conscious relationship with both food and medicine. You'll learn how to create sacred spaces for healing, understand the role of mindfulness in digestive health, and discover ways to honor both your body's wisdom and the benefits of modern medicine. Studies on the gut microbiome have shown that our emotional relationship with food and medicine can significantly impact their effectiveness.

As we explore these concepts, you'll discover how small shifts in awareness can lead to significant improvements in your digestive health and overall wellbeing. Whether you're dealing with medication-related digestive issues, seeking to enhance your body's natural healing capacity, or simply wanting to develop a more mindful approach to eating, this chapter offers practical tools and gentle guidance for your journey, grounded in both ancient wisdom and modern science.

Before we begin this exploration, take a moment to acknowledge your own wisdom. Your body holds deep intelligence, shaped by decades of experience, and by learning to listen more closely, you can create a more harmonious relationship with both food and medicine. Let this chapter be your guide in bridging the gap between modern medical knowledge and your body's innate healing wisdom.

Gut-Healing Awareness and Eating with Intention

Eating is more than just fuel—it's a form of communication. Every meal is an opportunity to either support healing or trigger imbalance. According to *The Journal of Clinical Investigation* and research from Harvard's School of Public Health, *how* you eat is just as important as *what* you eat. Your emotional state, eating environment, and even the timing of your meal can significantly influence your gut bacteria, enzyme production, and nutrient absorption.

The foundation of gut healing awareness begins with understanding the body's natural rhythms. Research from the Department of Neuroscience at the University of Wisconsin has demonstrated that our digestive system functions best when we eat in alignment with our circadian cycles. This means creating regular mealtimes and giving our bodies enough time to properly digest and absorb nutrients between meals.

Creating a healing environment for eating doesn't require anything fancy—just small, intentional changes. Start by selecting a quiet, calm space for your meals, free from screens and work distractions. Studies show that eating while stressed or distracted can reduce your digestive enzyme production by as much as 60%. A simple practice like taking three slow, deep breaths before your meal can activate your parasympathetic nervous system—your body's "rest and digest" mode—help optimize digestion and support gut healing.

Daily Practice

Before your next meal, light a candle, take three deep breaths, and say: "I nourish my body with awareness and intention."
Observe how your body responds — not just during the meal but hours later.

Keep a simple journal noting not just what you eat but how you feel before, during, and after meals. This practice can help identify patterns and triggers that affect your gut health.

Remember that developing gut healing awareness is a journey, not a destination. Each meal provides an opportunity to tune into your body's signals and strengthen your connection to your digestive wisdom. Notice without judgment how different foods and eating environments affect your digestion, energy, and overall wellbeing.

The timing of our meals also plays a crucial role in gut healing. Research from the Department of Nutrition at Harvard School of Public Health shows that allowing adequate time between meals supports the migrating motor complex—our gut's natural cleaning system. Consider implementing a gentle 12-hour overnight fast, aligning with your body's natural repair and regeneration cycles.

Your goal isn't perfection but progress. Some days, you may find it easier to maintain mindful eating practices than others. Return to these practices with gentleness and compassion whenever you notice you've strayed. Each meal is a new opportunity to nourish your body with awareness and intention.

Your body holds ancient wisdom about what it needs to thrive. By developing gut healing awareness and eating with intention, you're not just improving your digestion—you're creating a foundation for vibrant health that supports every aspect of your wellbeing. Let each meal become a sacred moment of connection with your body's innate healing wisdom.

Rewriting the Story of Your Body: Medicine Without Resistance

The profound connections between our emotional relationship with medicine and its effectiveness in healing have been published in *the Journal of Clinical Investigation*. It demonstrates that our mindset about medical treatments can significantly influence their therapeutic outcomes. This understanding opens new possibilities for creating harmony between conventional medicine and our body's natural healing abilities.

The journey toward health often involves both medical support and our body's innate wisdom. Research shows that resistance to medical treatments can create additional stress, potentially impacting gut health and overall wellbeing. By developing a balanced perspective that honors both modern medical advances and natural healing processes, we can create a more effective path to wellness.

When we approach medicine with understanding rather than resistance, we create an environment that supports healing. Consider your current beliefs about medical treatments. Do they stem from past experiences, cultural influences, or perhaps misconceptions? Understanding the source of any resistance allows us to make more informed choices about our health care.

For many women over 50, the topic of medicine carries emotional weight — resistance, fear, or even shame. But as we move through this stage of life, it becomes essential to reframe how we view medical support. Emerging research in psychoneuroimmunology and clinical medicine shows that our mindset can influence how our bodies respond to treatment. When medication is taken with anxiety, guilt, or distrust, it may not be as effective. On the other hand, approaching it with calm, trust, and informed acceptance can enhance its benefits. Your beliefs don't just shape your thoughts—they shape your biology, too.

❀ Catherine's Journaling and Gratitude Practice ❀

Catherine, 64, struggled with this. "I hated taking my reflux pills," she admitted. "It made me feel like I'd failed my body." Through gentle journaling and daily gratitude practices, Catherine reframed medicine as an *act of love*, not defeat. Her symptoms eased, and her emotional energy lifted. "Now I thank my body for asking for help—and I thank the medicine for answering."

When we view medical treatments as allies in our healing journey rather than necessary evils, we may experience better outcomes and fewer side effects.

Building Understanding and Trust with Medicine

As we learn to build a respectful, balanced relationship with medicine, it's equally important to listen to the body's quiet signals—those subtle yet telling indicators that something deeper may be unfolding beneath the surface. Changes like ridges in the fingernails, thinning hair, dry or sagging skin, or dark urine and pale stools are not merely random quirks of aging. They can point to imbalances in liver function, gut health, or nutrient absorption. A white-coated tongue may suggest yeast overgrowth or digestive issues. Puffiness or sagging under the eyes could reflect lymphatic stagnation, kidney strain, or sluggish detoxification. Pale eyes or drooping eyelids might signal fatigue, anemia, or hormonal shifts.

These signs are not warnings to fear—but invitations to pay closer attention. Rather than brushing them aside or rushing to self-diagnose, this is the moment to bring in the wisdom of a trusted healthcare provider. Find someone who looks at the whole picture, who helps identify root causes rather than masking symptoms, and who guides you with compassion and clarity through personalized solutions.

True healing doesn't come from rejecting medicine—it comes from partnering with it. Ask questions, stay curious, and let your body's signals and your intuition work alongside expert insight. That's the power of integrative, empowered care.

- Schedule checkups with healthcare providers who respect your preferences
- Keep a symptom and treatment journal
- Ask about natural alternatives or complementary options
- See medicine as part of a team — not the enemy

Clear communication with healthcare providers forms the foundation of effective treatment. Research shows that patients who actively engage in their medical care often experience better outcomes. This includes being honest about concerns, asking questions about treatments, and sharing experiences with natural remedies or lifestyle changes.

Building Healthcare Partnership

- Prepare questions before medical appointments
- Keep a symptom and treatment journal
- Share your goals and concerns openly
- Request explanations in terms you understand
- Discuss the integration of natural approaches

Creating a personal wellness team might include both conventional and holistic practitioners. This could mean having a primary care physician who understands your interest in natural approaches alongside practitioners who support your overall wellness goals. The key is finding providers who respect your desire for an integrated approach to health.

A health timeline that includes both medical treatments and natural healing practices would be good record-keeping and easy access for references. This visual representation can help you see how different approaches complement each other and contribute to your overall wellbeing. Remember that rewriting your story with medicine isn't about erasing the past – it's about creating a new narrative that serves your highest good.

Our relationship with medicine and aging is often layered with beliefs, hopes, and even resistance. Taking a moment to explore what you truly believe about healing—whether from your body, nature, or modern medicine—can offer powerful insights. Ask yourself: Where do I feel hesitation, and what story lies beneath it? Healing becomes more holistic when we choose to honor both our body's inner wisdom and the medical support we receive.

A simple daily practice can help align intention with action: before taking any medication or supplement, pause, place your hand on your heart, and say, *"I welcome this support for my healing journey."* This small ritual transforms the act from routine to sacred, reminding you that healing is not just about what you take, but the energy and mindset you bring to it.

Your Emotional Relationship with Healing

Your gut and brain are connected by the gut-brain axis — a two-way communication line powered by hormones, nerves, and microbes. If your mind is anxious, your gut feels it. If your gut is inflamed, your thoughts can fog.

This connection goes deeper when it comes to how we feel about our healing journey. Studies confirm that emotional stress affects digestion and medication absorption. But when you bring awareness to your inner landscape, healing deepens.

The way we feel about our medications and treatments profoundly influences their effectiveness in supporting our wellness journey. Research published in *the Journal of Clinical Investigation* demonstrates that our emotional response to medicine can significantly impact its therapeutic benefits. This understanding becomes particularly relevant as we navigate health changes after fifty, where multiple medications or treatments might become part of our daily routine.

Consider your immediate emotional response when taking medication or following treatment protocols. Do you approach them with acceptance and gratitude for their supporting role in your wellness journey? Or do you notice resistance, worry, or even resentment? These aren't just passing thoughts – studies show they can influence how our bodies respond to treatment.

Psychoneuroimmunology reveals that our emotional state while taking medicine affects its absorption and effectiveness. When we approach our treatments with tension or resistance, we may inadvertently create barriers to their full therapeutic potential. Conversely, when we cultivate a mindset of acceptance and partnership with our medications, we support their intended benefits.

Emotional Healing Tools

- Start a "Medicine + Mood" journal
- Practice 3 deep breaths before meals and meds
- Use loving affirmations
- Reflect on where emotional wounds may be causing resistance

Integration: Creating Harmony Between Wisdom and Support

You don't have to choose between medical treatment and inner wisdom. You can honor both — and thrive in doing so. Just like Eleanor and Catherine, you are not just surviving — you're evolving.

Let each meal be a chance to connect. Let each treatment be a moment of care. Let each breath be a reminder: *your body is working with you, not against you.*

Our gut microbiome responds to emotional stress, potentially affecting how we metabolize medications. By cultivating a more positive emotional relationship with our treatments, we may enhance their effectiveness while supporting our overall gut health.

Creating harmony with medicine doesn't mean ignoring side effects or concerns. Instead, it means approaching these challenges with curiosity and openness, working collaboratively with healthcare providers to find solutions that honor both your physical and emotional wellbeing.

Your emotional relationship with medicine is an integral part of your healing journey. By bringing awareness, compassion, and intention to this relationship, you create space for deeper healing and more effective treatment outcomes. Remember, every step toward a more positive medicine relationship is a step toward better health and wellbeing. As we conclude this transformative exploration of mindful wellness and medicine integration, let the wisdom shared in this chapter continue to guide your journey. The delicate dance between modern medical support and your body's innate healing wisdom creates a foundation for lasting vitality. Through mindful awareness and conscious choices, you've discovered how to create harmony between these essential aspects of health

Core Integration Practices:

- Create peaceful rituals for both meals and medications
- Stay open, curious, and informed about your treatment choices
- Practice gratitude — for your body, your tools, your journey
- Keep honest conversations open with your healthcare team

The journey of transforming your relationship with food and medicine continues beyond these pages. Each meal becomes an opportunity for mindful nourishment, each treatment a chance to practice acceptance and trust. Your body holds profound wisdom, and modern medicine offers valuable support—together, they create a powerful partnership for healing.

Remember that this transformation unfolds gradually, one mindful choice at a time. Whether you're adjusting eating habits, exploring new treatments, or learning to trust your body's signals, each step forward strengthens your foundation for vibrant health.

Practice for Tomorrow

Begin your day with three conscious breaths before your first meal or medicine. Notice how this simple practice affects your experience. Let this awareness guide you toward choices that honor both your body's wisdom and medical support.

Recent research continues to validate the profound connection between mindful awareness and healing outcomes. Your journey toward integrated wellness supports not just your physical health, but your emotional and spiritual wellbeing as well.

As you close this chapter, celebrate how far you've come. Every mindful meal, every conscious breath, and every moment of acceptance builds your capacity for deeper healing.

Trust that your body knows how to heal while honoring the support available through medicine. This balance creates space for true transformation, allowing you to thrive in your golden years with grace, vitality, and wisdom.

Your next chapter awaits, but for now, rest in the knowledge that you're creating harmony between ancient wisdom and modern medicine—a powerful foundation for lasting health.

CHAPTER 4
The Stress-Gut Connection:
Balancing Cortisol for Better Health

Every time you feel butterflies in your stomach before an important event or lose your appetite during times of worry, you're experiencing firsthand the powerful connection between your stress levels and your digestive system. This remarkable relationship is governed by a complex network of hormones, particularly cortisol, which acts as both a protector and potential disruptor of your gut health, depending on how well you manage your daily stress levels.

A research published in *Current Opinion in Behavioral Sciences* reveals how this invisible yet potent relationship between stress and digestion profoundly shapes our daily health. For women over fifty, understanding this connection becomes increasingly crucial as hormonal changes can amplify stress responses, potentially disrupting both digestive function and emotional wellbeing.

Let's begin with a gentle reminder: "I nurture my body with peaceful awareness, knowing that each calm breath supports my digestive healing."

Scientific studies, including recent work by researchers Madison and Kiecolt-Glaser, demonstrate that this type of chronic stress can significantly alter gut function through elevated cortisol levels. These stress-induced shifts create a feedback loop: the more disrupted your gut becomes, the more emotional tension you may feel—fueling a cycle of discomfort that affects both body and mind. In this chapter, we'll explore practical ways to recognize and respond to stress-related digestive issues. You'll discover why your digestion might feel particularly sensitive during times of worry and more importantly, how to support your body's natural healing abilities through evidence-based stress-management techniques specifically designed for women in their golden years.

Through gentle yet effective strategies, you'll learn how to create your own stress-management toolkit that supports both emotional and digestive wellness. Whether you're dealing with occasional digestive discomfort or chronic stress-related symptoms, this chapter will guide you toward finding your unique path to balance.

🌸 Patricia and Maya's Journey 🌸

Consider Patricia's journey—at 62, this devoted grandmother found herself facing unprecedented digestive challenges after her husband's health scare. Despite being the family's rock, she noticed increasing bloating and irregular bowel movements that intensified every time she checked her phone for updates about her husband. Through mindful observation, Patricia realized she was holding her breath and tensing her belly without even noticing. Her body had been whispering for rest and gentleness.

Or take Maya, 59, a woman doing everything "right" on paper—clean eating, daily walks, probiotic supplements—but still struggling with stubborn bloating and fatigue. Her turning point came not from another supplement but from embracing small rituals of calm. Morning breathing practices and evening wind-down routines helped her nervous system unwind. Her body, finally feeling safe, began to respond. "I stopped fighting," she reflected. "I started listening."

These stories remind us that the missing piece in gut healing isn't always about food—it's about how we breathe, rest, and relate to stress.

In this chapter, you'll discover how to:

- Recognize stress-related digestive patterns
- Understand cortisol's role in the gut-brain connection
- Apply science-backed techniques to calm your nervous system
- Create daily rituals for resilience and rest

Together, we'll build a toolkit that supports not just your digestion but your joy, peace, and sense of inner balance.

Your journey to better gut health isn't just about what you eat—it's about how you live, breathe, and respond to life's challenges. As we explore the intricate dance between stress and digestion, you'll discover practical tools to support your body's natural healing abilities, helping you create lasting change in both your digestive health and overall wellbeing.

Understanding the Stress Response: How Cortisol Impacts Your Gut

When stress activates our body's alarm system, it triggers a cascade of hormonal changes designed to help us respond to perceived threats. At the center of this response is cortisol. While cortisol plays a vital role in our survival, its prolonged presence— especially in midlife and beyond—can undermine our digestive system's natural rhythm.

Recent insights from the field of psychoneuroimmunology reveal just how deeply chronic stress can affect gut health—slowing digestion, increasing gut permeability (known as "leaky gut"), reducing beneficial bacteria, and heightening inflammation. For women in their golden years, these effects may be amplified by hormonal changes already influencing digestion and nutrient absorption. But knowledge is power, and understanding this gut-stress connection opens the door to healing.

Simple practices like gentle breathing (inhale for 4, exhale for 6), starting the day with quiet time before screens, eating softer foods on stressful days, and taking peaceful post-meal walks can help regulate the nervous system and support digestion. A stress-digestion journal can also offer insight into how emotions manifest physically, allowing you to respond with compassion rather than control. These small, intentional choices can soothe both the gut and the mind—creating space for calm, clarity, and healing from the inside out.

Journal Prompt

Where do you feel stress in your body first? How does your digestion shift under stress? What soothes and grounds you?

Research by Badal et al. reveals that chronic stress can alter the gut microbiome within hours, highlighting the importance of developing effective stress management strategies. The good news is that our gut bacteria can show positive changes just as quickly when we implement stress-reduction techniques.

The Practical Implementation to Ongoing Wellness starts with small changes. Perhaps begin your day with three deep breaths before getting out of bed, or take a moment to consciously relax your shoulders and jaw before eating. Notice how your body responds to these moments of intentional calm.

Your stress response isn't your enemy—it's a protective mechanism that's trying to keep you safe. By understanding this relationship and responding with compassion, you can begin to create a more harmonious balance between your stress levels and gut health.

Even brief relaxation—like three deep breaths—has been shown to improve gut barrier function. These simple practices support both the microbiome and mood, gently rewiring your stress response.

Ask yourself: What one stress-management technique could I commit to this week that would support my digestive wellness? Remember, consistency with a simple practice often yields better results than attempting complex protocols sporadically.

As you move forward, focus on progress, not perfection. Your body has an innate wisdom—when we create conditions for balance, it knows how to heal and thrive. Each step toward managing stress is also a step toward better gut health, creating a foundation for lasting wellness in your golden years.

Signs of Stress-Related Digestive Issues in Women Over 50

Bodies often become more responsive—and more vulnerable—to the effects of stress. For many women over 50, stress doesn't just show up as tension or fatigue; it often whispers through the gut. Bloating, constipation, indigestion, or sudden appetite changes can all be subtle yet powerful signals that something deeper is unfolding.

Understanding how stress presents itself through your digestive system empowers you to respond early before symptoms escalate. These shifts are not random—they are your body's way of asking for care, calm, and support. By tuning into these cues, you open the door to more effective stress management and long-term gut wellness. Research shows that stress may manifest as:

- Bloating or trapped gas

- Constipation or sudden urgency Acid reflux
- Nausea, loss of appetite, or emotional eating
- Increased food sensitivities
- Disrupted gut sounds or sensations

Research by Madison and Kiecolt-Glaser demonstrates how these symptoms connect directly to the gut-brain axis, showing that addressing stress can significantly improve digestive function. For women over 50, hormonal changes can amplify these stress responses, making recognition of early warning signs particularly important.

🌷 Angela Learned to Catch the Signs 🌷

Angela, 63, noticed her symptoms flared before hosting family gatherings. With journaling, she identified a pattern: tightness in her throat and shallow breathing often preceded digestive upset. By honoring these signals, she learned how to respond before symptoms escalated.

When stress or discomfort feels overwhelming, a simple reset can help bring your body and mind back into balance. The Emergency Reset Protocol offers a gentle, grounding practice you can use anytime, anywhere. Begin by pausing and taking three deep, intentional breaths. Place your hand over your belly and softly affirm, *"I am safe. I am calm."*

This mindful touch signals safety to your nervous system. Then, sip warm water slowly to soothe your digestion and encourage relaxation. If possible, step outside for a brief walk—nature and movement together help shift your energy gently. These small actions may seem simple, but they can create a powerful ripple effect, calming the gut, steadying the breath, and reminding your body that it is supported, moment by moment.

Emergency Reset Protocol

- Pause
- Take three deep breaths
- Place your hand over your belly and say: "I am safe. I am calm."
- Sip warm water slowly
- If possible, take a short outdoor walk

Reflection Prompt

What emotions or situations tend to precede your digestive discomfort? How can you respond earlier, with care and kindness?

Research shows that the gut microbiome is highly sensitive and can respond to stress signals within just a few hours, often disrupting digestion, increasing inflammation, or shifting microbial balance. While this may sound alarming, it's also empowering—because the very same responsiveness means that calming practices can bring relief just as swiftly. Techniques like deep breathing, gentle movement, mindfulness, and emotional awareness can quickly signal safety to the nervous system, helping to restore digestive harmony. In essence, the gut listens—and when you offer it calm and care, it begins to rebalance and heal in real time.

Remember that these symptoms aren't just 'in your head' - they represent real physiological changes in your digestive system. When stress activates our fight-or-flight response, it can:

- Decrease digestive enzyme production
- Alter gut motility
- Reduce nutrient absorption
- Impact the gut microbiome composition
- Increase inflammation markers

Practical Stress Management Techniques for Gut Health

Understanding how stress impacts our gut health is important, but even more crucial is having practical techniques to manage that stress effectively. Research from Madison and Kiecolt-Glaser demonstrates that implementing stress management strategies can significantly improve gut microbiome health and digestive function, particularly for women over 50.

Managing stress effectively is one of the most powerful and loving gifts you can offer your gut. In our fast-paced lives, stress often becomes a silent disruptor—elevating cortisol, straining the nervous system, and disturbing the delicate balance of the gut microbiome. But science now confirms that when we consciously slow down and engage in calming practices, we don't just feel better emotionally—we initiate real physiological healing.

Mindful breathing, gentle movement, meditation, time in nature, and meaningful social connection are all proven to regulate cortisol levels and enhance microbial diversity in the gut. This diversity is not a minor detail—it's a cornerstone of overall health, supporting strong immunity, smooth digestion, hormone balance, and emotional resilience. Each intentional act of calm sends a message to your gut that it is safe, supported, and able to return to balance. Healing doesn't require perfection—it begins with presence and with choosing peace in the small, everyday moments that truly matter.

Through personal life experiences, I have discovered that evening relaxation practices can improve sleep quality, which in turn supports better gut health and stress resilience.

Always start small—because in healing, consistency matters more than intensity. Even five minutes of conscious breathing, gentle stretching, or a quiet walk can begin to calm your stress response and gently support your digestive system. These small acts may seem simple, but they speak volumes to your body, signaling safety and stability. As you develop these practices, tune in with curiosity. Notice how your body responds—what feels soothing, what feels strained—and adjust with kindness. Over time, these little moments of care become powerful habits that lay the foundation for lasting gut and emotional health.

Monitor your progress by keeping a simple journal noting:

- Energy levels
- Digestive comfort
- Stress triggers
- Effective coping strategies
- Sleep quality

Most importantly, approach these practices with self-compassion. Healing is not a race, and every small step you take is a meaningful act of self-care. Each day offers a new opportunity to nurture the powerful connection between your gut and brain, building resilience gently—one breath, one mindful choice at a time. As we conclude this exploration of the stress-gut connection, take a moment to reflect on the deep insights we've uncovered. Science continues to affirm what intuition already knows: our emotional wellbeing and digestive health are deeply intertwined. For women over 50, learning to understand and regulate the stress response isn't just helpful—it's essential for maintaining vibrant gut health, balanced hormones, and overall vitality. Trust in the wisdom of your body, and let each practice become a quiet declaration of healing from within.

Journal Reflection

What daily practice makes you feel most soothed? How could you make that a habit?

Chapter Conclusion: Integration & Inner Peace

Through the stories of Patricia, Maya, and Angela—and the research guiding us—we've discovered that managing stress is not just a mental health strategy but a digestive health necessity.

Key Takeaways

- Chronic stress impacts gut function, especially post-50
- Mindfulness, breathwork, and connection reduce cortisol and aid digestion
- Your gut responds quickly to emotional and environmental shifts
- Healing begins with awareness, not perfection

Reflection Questions

- What's one area of stress you could soften this week?
- Which calming ritual speaks most to your lifestyle?
- How will you support your gut through your next challenging moment?

This journey isn't about achieving perfect stress-free living—it's about building resilience and understanding. Your body isn't your enemy; it's your ally in healing. Each small step toward stress management is a step toward better gut health.

As you move forward, carry with you the knowledge that your stress response can be reset at any age. The research clearly shows that even small changes in how we manage stress can lead to significant improvements in gut health and overall wellbeing.

For now, rest in this truth: your calm is your medicine.

Your journey to vibrant health continues with every mindful moment you choose. Let your breath lead the way.

Practical Action

- Keep a daily symptom tracker noting food, mood, and stress levels
- Pause three times a day to scan your body for tension or unease
- Build awareness around how emotional states map to digestive changes

In the next chapter, we'll explore how to nourish your gut for natural weight balance and sustainable energy through gut healing and natural weight management, building on this foundation of stress awareness and mindful living.

Daily Affirmation

"With each mindful breath, I restore peace to my body, and my gut heals with ease."

CHAPTER 5
Eating and Resetting the Gut to Fire Up Metabolism for Natural Weight Management

"My body knows how to heal, and I trust its wisdom as I create new patterns of nourishment and care."

The journey to optimal health after fifty isn't about strict calorie counting or chasing the latest diet trends. It's more about working *with* your body—aligning your meals with its natural rhythms and nourishing your inner ecosystem with foods that support both gut healing and metabolic balance.

When we understand this powerful connection, we open the door to a renewed vitality—one that many women over 50 may have thought was out of reach. Like a well-tended garden, your gut and metabolism flourish when cared for consistently, with the right nutrients and a gentle, rhythmic approach to eating.

In this chapter, we'll explore how timing your meals, choosing gut-supportive foods, and creating sustainable eating patterns can gently reset your metabolism while healing your digestive system. This isn't about restriction or deprivation – it's about working in harmony with your body's natural wisdom to create lasting change.

Recent research highlighted in the journal *'Nutrients'* has shown that the timing of our meals plays a crucial role in maintaining metabolic health, particularly for women over 50. The study demonstrated that aligning eating patterns with our circadian rhythms can significantly improve gut function and metabolic efficiency.

Barbara's story perfectly illustrates this transformative journey. As a 57-year-old artist, she had spent decades caught in the cycle of yo-yo dieting, which had left both her gut health and metabolism compromised. Her habit of skipping breakfast and eating late into the evening while working on her paintings had created a pattern of digestive distress and unwanted weight gain. Through learning to align her eating patterns with her body's natural rhythms and incorporating nurturing, gut-healing foods, Barbara discovered that sustainable weight management came not from restriction but from nourishment.

Like Barbara, many women find themselves caught between conflicting advice about weight management after 50. The truth is, your body isn't failing you—it's asking for a different kind of care. When we honor our digestive system's needs and natural cycles, we create the foundation for both gut healing and metabolic balance.

Joan's experience further reinforces this wisdom. At 61, despite eating 'clean' and maintaining a regular exercise routine, she found herself stuck at a plateau. What she discovered was transformative—her gut was holding onto inflammation, not fat. By shifting her focus from restriction to nourishment—choosing warm, healing meals and embracing gut-supportive foods—Joan experienced changes she once thought were out of reach. Her body began to respond with renewed energy, comfort, and ease.

As we delve deeper into this chapter, you'll discover practical strategies for timing your meals, selecting foods that nurture both gut healing and metabolic health balance, and developing eating patterns that feel sustainable and joyful. Keep in mind this journey isn't about reaching a number on the scale – it's about creating lasting harmony between your gut and metabolism, allowing your body to find its natural balance.

Timing Matters:
Understanding Circadian Eating for Metabolic Health

Think of your digestive system as an orchestra. When each section (enzymes, gut bacteria, metabolism) plays in rhythm, your body functions in harmony. But when meals are mistimed—like eating late at night or skipping breakfast—it disrupts that internal melody.

Think of your digestive system as an orchestra performing a daily connection. Just as musicians need precise timing to create harmony, your body's metabolic processes require specific timing to function optimally. Your gut microbiome, digestive enzymes, and metabolic hormones all follow this natural rhythm known as your circadian cycle.

Eating in alignment with these natural patterns can significantly improve digestion, metabolism, and overall health. A study in *the journal Nutrients* demonstrated that women over 50 who aligned their eating schedule with their circadian rhythm experienced better blood sugar control, improved sleep quality, and more efficient digestion.

Scientific research supports this: eating your main meals earlier in the day, ideally when the sun is at its peak, improves digestion, blood sugar balance, and even sleep. Studies also show that women over 50 benefits greatly from a 12–14 hour overnight fasting window.

Practical Implementation Guide

- Start the day with warm lemon water to gently awaken digestion
- Eat your first meal within 2–3 hours of waking

- Make lunch your largest meal between 12–2 PM
- Finish dinner 2–3 hours before bedtime
- Allow 12–14 hours of overnight fasting for gut rest

🌸 Carol's Insight 🌸

Carol, at 64, shifted her meals earlier and noticed improved energy, reduced bloating, and better sleep—without changing what she ate, only *when* she ate it.

Journal Prompt

When do you typically eat your meals? How do you feel afterward? What one small change could you try this week to better align with your body's rhythm?

Understanding your natural eating patterns is the first step toward creating sustainable change. This isn't about rigid rules but rather about gently guiding your body back to its natural rhythm. Start with one small adjustment, perhaps moving dinner 30 minutes earlier or establishing a consistent breakfast time.

Studies have shown that eating your main meal when the sun is highest (typically between 12-2 PM) supports optimal nutrient absorption and metabolic function. This timing aligns perfectly with your body's natural enzymatic activity and can help reduce evening cravings and improve sleep quality.

Simple Strategy for Success

Begin by tracking your meals for one week without making changes. Notice when you eat and how you feel afterward. Then, gradually shift one meal at a time closer to the recommended windows. This gentle approach allows your body to adapt without resistance.

The flexibility is key - some days may require different timing, and that's perfectly normal. The goal is to work with your body's rhythm most of the time while allowing for life's natural variations. Your body will thank you with improved digestion, more stable energy, and better overall metabolic health.

Gut-Healing Foods and Meal Patterns for Women Over 50

Drawing from a research published in *the journal 'Nutrients,'* we now understand that specific foods and eating patterns can significantly support gut healing and metabolic health in women over 50. The research highlights how certain nutrients and compounds work synergistically to repair and maintain digestive wellness while supporting healthy aging.

The gut is like a garden—it thrives with consistency and the right nutrients. Research published in *Nutrients* and the *Journal of Nutrition* highlights several key foods that support a healthy microbiome, reduce inflammation, and support weight regulation.

Top Gut-Healing Foods

- **Fermented foods:** sauerkraut, kimchi, kefir, yogurt
- **Prebiotic fibers:** garlic, onions, leeks, asparagus
- **Anti-inflammatory proteins:** wild-caught fish, legumes, bone broth
- **Polyphenol-rich foods:** berries, dark greens, herbs
- **Fiber-rich vegetables**: sweet potatoes, carrots, beets
- **Digestive spices:** turmeric, ginger, cinnamon

Sample Gut-Healing Meal Pattern

- **Breakfast:** Warm lemon water → protein (eggs or smoothie) + fiber-rich fruit
  - Start with warm lemon water
  - Include easily digestible protein
  - Add fiber-rich fruits or vegetables
  - Consider probiotic-rich foods

- **Lunch (largest meal):** Quality protein + colorful veg + fermented food
  - o Begin with bitter greens or fermented vegetables
  - o Include quality protein and healthy fats
  - o Add a variety of colorful vegetables
  - o Incorporate healing herbs and spices
- **Dinner:** Cooked vegetables + gentle herbs + small portion of healthy fats
  - o Keep portions moderate
  - o Focus on well-cooked, easily digestible foods
  - o Include gentle herbs for digestion
  - o Consider ending with ginger or peppermint tea

Practical Tip

Start with one change—perhaps a teaspoon of sauerkraut at lunch or bone broth before dinner. Your body's feedback will guide you.

Emotional Integration

Let go of judgment around "good" or "bad" eating days. Each meal is a new opportunity to nourish and reconnect.

Research published in the Journal of Nutrition reveals that women over 50 who regularly consume fermented foods experience improved digestive function and enhanced immune response. The key is introducing these foods gradually and observing how your body responds.

A study focused on gut microbiome health demonstrated that consuming a variety of fiber-rich vegetables supports the growth of beneficial bacteria like Akkermansia muciniphila, which plays a crucial role in maintaining gut barrier function and metabolic health.

Additional supportive meal patterns are equally important. Research suggests that following these guidelines can enhance digestion and nutrient absorption:

- Begin meals with bitter greens or fermented vegetables to stimulate digestion
- Include protein and fiber at each meal to support stable blood sugar
- Allow 3-4 hours between meals for proper digestion
- Incorporate healing herbs and spices like turmeric, ginger, and cinnamon

Many of the gut-healing foods you may already include in your diet—such as leafy greens, cruciferous vegetables, and fermented foods—do more than support digestion; they also play a vital role in liver function and microbial balance. Fiber-rich plants and bitter greens like dandelion or arugula stimulate bile production, which helps the liver break down fats and eliminate toxins more efficiently. Fermented foods like kimchi, kefir, and sauerkraut introduce beneficial bacteria that not only aid digestion but also create a gut environment where powerful microbes like *Akkermansia muciniphila* can thrive. This particular bacterium helps maintain the integrity of the gut lining and has been linked to reduced inflammation and improved metabolic health. As you tune into how your body responds to these foods—especially fermented ones—you may begin to notice subtle shifts in energy, digestion, and even mood. This week, consider a gentle addition: a scoop of sauerkraut with lunch, a handful of steamed greens, or a warm cup of lemon water before breakfast. These small steps support a powerful inner ecosystem where your liver, gut, and beneficial bacteria work in harmony to restore and revitalize your health.

Start by adding one new gut-healing food each week. Perhaps begin with a small portion of sauerkraut with lunch or incorporating cooked bitter greens with dinner. Listen to your body's response and adjust accordingly.

Remember, healing isn't about perfection – it's about progress and consistency. Your digestive system will respond best to gentle, gradual changes rather than dramatic overhauls. Focus on adding nourishing foods rather than restricting, allowing your gut microbiome to adapt and thrive naturally.

Your journey to gut healing is unique, and what works for one person may need adjustment for another. Pay attention to how different foods and eating patterns affect your digestion, energy levels, and overall wellbeing. Through mindful observation and gentle implementation, you'll discover the combination that best supports your body's healing process.

Building a Sustainable Eating Strategy for Long-Term Weight Management

Sustainable weight balance after 50 stems from honoring your gut, supporting metabolic rhythms, and creating habits that feel *natural*. Restrictive plans fail because they ignore the body's wisdom and your unique lifestyle.

When we think about gut-healing foods, imagine your digestive system as a garden that needs specific nutrients to flourish. Recent studies have shown that incorporating certain foods can actively support the growth of beneficial gut bacteria while reducing inflammation and supporting digestive repair.

Sustainable weight management, especially for women over 50, isn't about strict diets or willpower—it's about creating a nourishing rhythm that supports your body's natural balance. A gut-friendly approach begins with consistent meal timing, including periods of gentle overnight fasting to allow your digestive system to rest and reset. Building balanced plates with protein, fiber, healthy fats, and complex carbs keeps blood sugar stable and cravings in check. But what's on your plate is only part of the story.

Mindful eating—slowing down, savoring each bite, and expressing gratitude—helps your body better recognize when you are full and satisfied. Emotional healing also plays a vital role: acknowledging past struggles with dieting, releasing shame, and identifying stress-eating triggers pave the way for real transformation. And never underestimate the power of social connection—sharing meals with people who uplift you can turn eating into a joyful, healing ritual. When these elements come together, weight management becomes less about control and more about harmony—honoring your gut, your emotions, and your whole self.

Martha, at 64, joined a weekly cooking circle that not only improved her meals but also strengthened her joy and connection.

Simple Implementation Steps

- **Start small:** One new food or timing adjustment per week
- **Observe:** Keep a journal on digestion, mood, and energy
- **Adjust:** Honor your body's feedback and tweak accordingly
- **Celebrate:** Every shift, no matter how small is a step toward healing

Research shows that successful long-term weight management comes from making small, consistent changes that become natural parts of your daily routine. Focus on adding nourishing practices rather than restricting or eliminating foods.

Think of your strategy as a flexible framework rather than a rigid plan. This allows for adaptation while maintaining the core principles that support your health. Consider keeping a simple journal to track what works best for you and adjust accordingly.

Understand that sustainable change happens gradually. Your body needs time to adjust to new patterns and heal from previous imbalances. Trust this process and celebrate small improvements along the way.

Reflection Questions

- What meal patterns feel natural and energizing?
- What's one nourishing habit you can add this week?
- Who can you share your journey with for support and joy?

By focusing on sustainability rather than quick fixes, you create lasting change that supports both your gut health and natural weight management. This approach honors your body's wisdom while creating patterns that enhance your vitality for years to come. As we close this enlightening chapter on resetting metabolism and nurturing gut health, we recognize the profound connection between eating patterns, digestive wellness, and sustainable weight management. The research is clear—our bodies respond best to gentle, consistent practices that honor natural rhythms and support healing from within.

Through the stories of Barbara and Joan, we've seen how aligning meals with our circadian rhythm and focusing on gut-supportive foods can transform not just our digestion but our entire relationship with eating and wellness. Their experiences remind us that lasting change comes not from restriction but from understanding and working with our body's innate wisdom.

Chapter Summary: The Rhythm of Healing

True transformation isn't about the scale—it's about harmony. Aligning your meals with your body's rhythm, choosing foods that nourish, and embracing joy in eating are the real secrets to vibrant health.

Core Takeaways

- Eat in sync with your circadian rhythm
- Focus on gut-healing foods and gentle patterns
- Develop sustainable habits rooted in compassion
- Prioritize emotional wellness and social connection

In the next chapter, we'll explore how your microbiome shapes immunity and vitality. For now, trust that your body is capable of profound healing—one nourishing moment at a time.

Be focused on implementing what resonates most deeply from these teachings. Trust that your body will guide you toward what it needs most, one mindful meal at a time.

Let the wisdom you've gained here be your foundation as you continue building sustainable patterns that support both your gut health and metabolism. Through consistent, gentle practices and mindful attention to your body's signals, you're creating lasting change that will serve you well into your vibrant future.

Your healing journey is unique, and it's unfolding exactly as it should. Trust this process, celebrate small victories, and know that every step forward, no matter how small, is progress worth honoring.

CHAPTER 6
Your Microbiome Blueprint:
Building Immunity and Vitality

"I nurture my inner ecosystem with love and awareness, knowing it supports my vibrant health and natural immunity."

Within your digestive system lives a vast community of microorganisms that rivals the complexity of an ancient forest, each species playing a crucial role in maintaining your health and vitality. This microscopic ecosystem, known as your microbiome, holds the key to not just your digestive wellness, but also your immune strength, energy levels, and even your emotional resilience as you navigate your golden years.

"Your microbiome is your silent protector—when it thrives, you do too." Think of your microbiome as a vibrant garden where each beneficial bacterium plays a vital role in your overall health and vitality. Just as a garden needs the right balance of nutrients, water, and care to flourish, your internal ecosystem requires mindful attention and nourishment to support your immune system and maintain your natural vitality after 50.

Recent scientific research has revealed fascinating insights into how this microscopic community influences everything from our immune response to our emotional well-being. Studies published in journals such as *Nutrients*, *Current Biology*, and *Journal of Nutrition* show that a diverse and balanced microbiome enhances our ability to fight infections, regulate inflammation, and even support cognitive function. These findings are especially relevant for women over 50, as age-related changes in hormones and metabolism can disrupt gut balance.

The relationship between our microbiome and immune system is particularly intriguing. Research has shown that beneficial gut bacteria produce essential compounds that help regulate our immune response, reduce inflammation, and strengthen our body's natural defense mechanisms. These microscopic allies work tirelessly to maintain the delicate balance that keeps us healthy and resilient.

Maintaining this internal garden requires understanding and patience. Like any ecosystem, it responds to the care and attention we provide. Simple daily choices - from the foods we eat to how we manage stress - can either nurture or challenge our microbiome's delicate balance. The good news is that our gut bacteria are remarkably responsive to positive changes, even as we age.

In this chapter, we'll explore practical strategies for building and maintaining a healthy gut ecosystem. You'll learn about the foods that nourish beneficial bacteria, understand the signs of microbiome imbalance, and discover how to support your body's natural defence systems through simple, sustainable practices.

Your microbiome is resilient and responsive at any age. When provided with the right environment and nourishment, it has a remarkable ability to rebalance and regenerate, supporting your health and vitality in countless ways. Let's begin this journey of discovery together, exploring how to cultivate your internal garden for optimal health and immunity.

🌹 Grace's Story: A Journey of Immune Renewal 🌹

Grace, a 68-year-old retired librarian, once prided herself on her good health. But after a tough winter filled with colds and missed book club meetings, she felt depleted. Despite eating what she believed was a healthy diet, she lacked diversity in her food choices. By gradually introducing fermented foods like sauerkraut and yogurt, adding leafy greens, and experimenting with fiber-rich vegetables, Grace rebuilt her gut ecosystem. Four months later, she not only felt more resilient, but she also began leading her own fermentation workshops, reconnecting with joyful traditions.

Understanding Your Microbiome: The Foundation of Immune Health After 50

Recent studies confirm that the trillions of microorganisms in your gut form a sophisticated defense network.

Your microbiome acts as a living shield, creating what scientists refer to as a 'barrier effect.' These beneficial bacteria coat your intestinal lining, forming a protective barrier that helps determine what enters your bloodstream and what gets eliminated. This becomes especially crucial after 50, when natural changes in gut permeability can affect how your body responds to potential threats.

Research shows that specific beneficial bacteria, like Akkermansia muciniphila and Clostridium butyricum, play vital roles in maintaining this protective barrier. These microscopic allies produce compounds that help repair and strengthen your intestinal lining while training your immune cells to respond appropriately to various challenges.

The communication between your microbiome and immune system is remarkably sophisticated. Beneficial bacteria produce short-chain fatty acids, particularly butyrate, which serves as both fuel for your gut cells and a powerful anti-inflammatory compound. They also help regulate the production of antimicrobial substances and influence the development and function of your immune cells.

Your microbiome's influence extends beyond basic immunity. Studies indicate that a diverse gut ecosystem helps modulate inflammation throughout your body, supports the absorption of essential nutrients, and even influences how your body responds to stress. This becomes particularly relevant after 50, when maintaining balanced inflammation levels becomes increasingly important for overall health.

Your gut microbiome is more than just a collection of bacteria—it's a dynamic immune ally working around the clock to protect and nourish your body. One of its most vital roles is producing short-chain fatty acids (SCFAs), such as butyrate, which help regulate inflammation and maintain immune responses in check.

These compounds also strengthen the gut lining, preventing harmful substances from leaking into the bloodstream—a process known as reducing gut permeability. Beyond physical barriers, the microbiome plays a teaching role, educating immune cells to distinguish between friend and foe, thus preventing overreactions that lead to chronic inflammation or autoimmune issues. It also supports the absorption of essential nutrients such as zinc, vitamin D, and antioxidants, which are crucial for immune defense, tissue repair, and overall vitality. When your gut microbiome is nourished and diverse, it acts as a frontline guardian—calmly coordinating your immune system with wisdom and precision.

Signs of a Balanced Microbiome

- Regular, comfortable digestion
- Steady energy levels
- Emotional resilience and clear thinking
- Fewer seasonal illnesses
- Healthy skin and stable weight

Reflection Prompt

What signals does your body give when your digestion is happy and balanced? What changes help you feel most supported from within?

Nourishing Your Gut Garden: Foods and Practices That Support Beneficial Bacteria

Growing scientific evidence reveals that nourishing your gut microbiome requires more than just eating healthy—it's about creating an environment where beneficial bacteria can thrive. Research published in Nutrition Reviews highlights how specific dietary compounds, called polyphenols, act as prebiotics that selectively feed beneficial gut bacteria while discouraging harmful ones.

These polyphenols found abundantly in colorful fruits, vegetables, and herbs, work synergistically with your gut bacteria to produce compounds that reduce inflammation and support immune function. Studies show that women over 50, in particular, benefit from the regular consumption of polyphenol-rich foods, as they help counteract age-related changes in gut bacterial diversity.

Your beneficial gut bacteria need specific nutrients and care to flourish:

Top Gut-Nourishing Foods

- **Polyphenol-rich foods**: colorful berries, dark leafy greens, herbs
- **Fermented foods**: sauerkraut, kimchi, kefir, yogurt
- **Prebiotic foods**: garlic, onions, asparagus, Jerusalem artichokes

- **Resistant starches**: green bananas, cooked and cooled potatoes, use potatoes that were boiled and refrigerated overnight
- **Soluble fiber**: oats, legumes, carrots, beets

Food Prep & Eating Practices

- Soak legumes/grains before cooking for 6-8 hours and change the water a few times.
- Chew thoroughly and eat slowly
- Avoid overcooking vegetables to preserve nutrients
- Create a peaceful, tech-free eating environment

Signs Your Gut Garden is Thriving

- Consistent bowel movements
- Reduced sugar cravings
- Better mood and sleep quality
- Clearer skin and brighter eyes

Practical Tip

Gradually increase fiber and fermented foods. Start with a tablespoon of sauerkraut daily or try one new vegetable each week. Use a food-mood journal to track your response.

The timing of your meals plays a crucial role in maintaining a healthy balance of gut bacteria. Studies in Cell Host & Microbe demonstrate that our gut microbes follow daily rhythms, suggesting that regular meal timing helps optimize their beneficial activities. This becomes especially important after 50, when digestive patterns may naturally shift.

Fiber diversity emerges as another key factor in maintaining gut bacterial health. Research indicates that consuming 30 different plant foods weekly provides the variety of fibers and nutrients needed to support a diverse microbiome. This doesn't mean eating

30 different foods daily—rather, aim to incorporate various plant foods throughout your week.

When introducing new gut-supporting foods, start gradually to avoid overwhelming your digestive system. Begin with small portions of fermented foods like sauerkraut or kimchi, perhaps a tablespoon with meals, and slowly increase as your body adjusts. Similarly, when increasing fiber intake, do so progressively while ensuring adequate hydration.

Creating a sustainable approach to nourishing your gut garden involves finding balance rather than pursuing perfection. Focus on incorporating a variety of whole, minimally processed foods while honoring your body's unique needs and responses. Remember that small, consistent changes often yield better results than dramatic dietary overhauls.

Consider keeping a simple food and symptom diary as you explore new gut-nourishing foods and practices. This can help you identify patterns and understand which choices best support your unique microbiome. The goal isn't to create restrictions but rather to discover which foods and practices help your internal garden flourish.

Remember that your gut microbiome is remarkably resilient and responsive to positive changes at any age. By providing the right environment and nourishment, you support these beneficial bacteria in their vital work of maintaining your health and vitality. Each meal becomes an opportunity to tend to your internal garden, supporting the delicate balance that contributes to your overall wellbeing.

The Microbiome-Immunity Connection: Building Resilience Through Gut Health

Research published in recent scientific journals reveals an intricate dance between our gut microbiome and immune system that becomes increasingly important as we age. This partnership, far more sophisticated than previously understood, plays a crucial role in maintaining our health and resilience after 50.

Affirmation

"I honor the profound connection between my gut and immune system, nurturing both to create lasting resilience and vitality."

The gut microbiome acts as a sophisticated training ground for our immune cells. Studies show that beneficial bacteria help educate our immune system, teaching it to differentiate between harmful invaders and beneficial substances. This education process remains active throughout our lives, though it requires more conscious support as we age.

Evidence from recent research demonstrates how specific gut bacteria produce compounds called short-chain fatty acids (SCFAs) that help regulate inflammation and support immune function. These SCFAs, particularly butyrate, strengthen the gut barrier and help prevent unwanted substances from entering our bloodstream. They also communicate directly with immune cells, helping to maintain a balanced inflammatory response throughout the body.

The connection between gut health and immune resilience becomes particularly relevant for women over 50. Natural changes in hormones can affect both gut barrier function and immune response, making it essential to support this delicate partnership actively. Research indicates that maintaining a diverse microbiome helps counteract these age-related changes, supporting both digestive health and immune function.

Your gut barrier is your body's frontline defender—acting as a vigilant gatekeeper between your internal systems and the outside world. When supported by beneficial bacteria, this barrier remains strong and selective, preventing harmful substances from slipping through and triggering unnecessary immune responses. But when the gut barrier becomes compromised, it can allow unwanted intruders to pass, leading to chronic inflammation and a weakened immune system over time. Signs of a healthy gut-immune partnership include:

- Balanced immune responses without overreaction
- Quick recovery from occasional challenges
- Stable energy levels throughout the day
- Clear, comfortable digestion
- Resilient mood and emotional balance

Resilience isn't just a mindset—it's a biological process deeply rooted in the health of your gut. Your microbiome and immune system form a powerful partnership, constantly working together to keep you balanced, energized, and protected. Supporting this vital connection begins with *nutrient-dense foods* rich in immune-boosting compounds like antioxidants, fiber, and healthy fats that nourish both your body and beneficial gut bacteria.

Consistent sleep allows your gut and immune system to restore overnight, while mindful stress management—through breathing, journaling, or quiet reflection—calms the nervous system and supports microbial harmony. Gentle, regular movement, such as walking or stretching, encourages circulation and gut motility while hydrating with clean water helps flush toxins and maintain cellular health. Together, these practices don't just support digestion—

they build a resilient internal ecosystem that empowers you to face life's challenges with strength, grace, and vitality.

Recent studies highlight the importance of specific nutrients in supporting both gut and immune health. Polyphenols, found in colorful fruits and vegetables, help feed beneficial bacteria while supporting immune function. Zinc, vitamin D, and vitamin C play crucial roles in maintaining both gut barrier integrity and immune cell function.

The gut-immune connection also influences our emotional wellbeing. Research shows that a balanced microbiome helps regulate the production of neurotransmitters that affect mood and stress response. This emotional resilience becomes particularly important after 50, as stress can significantly impact both digestive and immune function.

Understanding this connection helps explain why digestive issues often coincide with increased susceptibility to illness. When our gut microbiome is imbalanced, it affects our immune system's ability to respond effectively to challenges. Conversely, supporting our gut health through diet and lifestyle choices helps build natural resilience.

For women over 50, gut-immune harmony becomes more important due to:

- Increased gut permeability from hormonal shifts
- Greater susceptibility to immune imbalance
- Emotional sensitivity influenced by gut-brain neurotransmitters

🌹 Linda's Story: Restoring Resilience 🌹

Linda, 65, faced recurring respiratory infections despite eating well. She discovered past antibiotics and chronic stress had compromised her microbiome. With a daily routine of probiotic foods, gratitude journaling, and sleep hygiene, she restored balance. Over time, her immune system bounced back, and her energy levels returned.

Final Reflections: Tending Your Inner Garden

Your microbiome is a powerful, responsive ally in your journey toward resilience, immunity, and energy after 50. Through mindful eating, daily rhythms, and nurturing practices, you can support this inner ecosystem in ways that bring profound healing.

Key Takeaways

- Align your meals and sleep with the circadian rhythm
- Embrace plant diversity and probiotic foods
- Start small, stay consistent, and observe your body
- Cultivate a calm internal and external environment

Journal Reflection

- What practice from this chapter feels most supportive right now?
- How does your inner ecosystem respond to changes in routine?
- What small habit will you begin this week?

Cherish that your body already holds the wisdom to heal. Each mindful step you take waters the seeds of lifelong vitality.

In the next chapter, we'll explore how to transform your kitchen into a sanctuary for gut healing, making it easier than ever to support your microbiome through delicious, nourishing meals.

Stay tuned and keep nurturing your inner garden with love, patience, and trust.

CHAPTER 7
The Healing Kitchen: Simple Foods
for Gut Wellness and Metabolism Reset Plan

*"I prepare my food with love and attention,
creating meals that nourish and heal my body."*

Your kitchen is more than just a place to prepare meals—it's a sanctuary where healing begins and vibrant health takes root. Within these walls, simple ingredients transform into powerful medicine, supporting your gut health and metabolism through time-tested wisdom combined with modern nutritional science.

Here, the simple act of preparing a meal becomes a quiet ritual— one that nourishes not just the body but the soul. It's in the slicing of fresh vegetables, the simmering of a stew, or the careful fermentation of ingredients that we reconnect with our health in the most intimate way.

Recent research published in the *Journal of Nutrition* affirms that how we prepare our food significantly impacts its ability to support our gut microbiome and overall metabolic health. Studies also show that traditional cooking methods, such as slow cooking and fermentation, enhance nutrient bioavailability while reducing digestive stress—a critical factor for women over 50.

Martha's Simplified Kitchen

Martha's journey illustrates that healing doesn't require complicated protocols or expensive ingredients. Like many women in their golden years, she discovered that returning to basics—

wholesome ingredients, mindful preparation, and time-honored methods—brought her renewed energy and digestive comfort. Through simplifying her approach, she transformed her kitchen into a healing space filled with ease, intention, and joy.

This chapter offers a practical, evidence-based roadmap to help you do the same. You'll learn how to stock your kitchen with essential tools and ingredients, apply gentle cooking methods that preserve nutrients, and plan meals aligned with your body's natural rhythms. With each step, you'll build a healing kitchen that supports both digestive wellness and metabolic balance.

Sometimes, the most profound healing comes not from what we add to our kitchens but from what we simplify and make space for.

For Martha, this simplification led to a deeper understanding of her body's needs. Her story teaches us that when we clear away the confusion and return to basics, our bodies often respond with renewed vitality. This approach is supported by recent studies showing that consistent, simple dietary practices often yield better results than complex, hard-to-maintain protocols.

As we explore the practical aspects of creating a healing kitchen, remember that your kitchen is not just a room – it's a powerful catalyst for transformation in your gut health journey. Every meal prepared with awareness becomes an opportunity to support your body's natural healing abilities and reset your metabolism, a concept increasingly supported by research in chronobiology and digestive health.

Essential Kitchen Tools and Ingredients for Gut Health

Creating an effective healing kitchen starts with having the right tools and ingredients. Behavioral psychology research confirms that when healthy items are visible and accessible, we make more nourishing choices consistently. Let's explore the essential items that can transform your kitchen into a sanctuary of gut health.

Core Kitchen Tools

- Large stock pot (for broths and soups)
- Glass storage containers
- Quality blender
- Mason jars (for fermentation and storage)
- Fine-mesh strainer (for teas and infusions)
- Wooden cutting boards and sharp knives

Tempered Glass and stainless steel cutting boards are preferable to plastic for minimizing harmful bacteria and endocrine disruptors. Each tool becomes part of your daily ritual, transforming food preparation into a healing experience.

Modern research in food science confirms that the materials we use for cooking and storage can significantly impact our gut health. Glass and wood materials, for instance, harbor fewer harmful bacteria compared to plastic alternatives, making them ideal for a healing kitchen environment

Essential Pantry Staples

- Healing herbs: ginger, turmeric, peppermint
- High-quality sea salt
- Raw apple cider vinegar
- Extra virgin olive oil (rich in polyphenols)
- Fiber-rich grains: quinoa, oats, brown rice
- Dried legumes: lentils, chickpeas

Fresh Ingredients to Keep On Hand

- Leafy greens (kale, spinach)
- Fermented foods (sauerkraut, yogurt, kimchi)

- Prebiotic vegetables (onions, garlic, leeks)
- Fresh herbs and citrus fruits
- Ginger and turmeric root

Keep your kitchen organized, clean, and calming. Add a plant, inspirational quote, or candle to imbue your space with positive energy. Remember, your kitchen is a healing sanctuary.

When selecting these items, quality matters more than quantity. Research published in the Journal of Nutrition has demonstrated that organic, minimally processed ingredients often contain higher levels of beneficial compounds that support gut health.

Fresh Ingredients for Gut Healing

Keep these fresh items on hand when possible:

- Leafy greens: kale, spinach, Swiss chard (rich in polyphenols)
- Fermented foods: sauerkraut, kimchi, natural yogurt
- Prebiotic-rich vegetables: garlic, onions, leeks
- Fresh herbs: parsley, cilantro, basil
- Ginger and turmeric root
- Citrus fruits: lemons, limes (support digestion)
- Fiber-rich vegetables: carrots, beets, sweet potatoes

Recent studies have shown that incorporating a variety of these fresh ingredients provides diverse nutrients and compounds that support a healthy gut microbiome. The key is to choose seasonal items, when possible, as they typically offer optimal nutritional value.

The organization of your healing kitchen matters as much as its contents. Keep frequently used items easily accessible, creating an environment that encourages healthy cooking. Research in behavioral psychology suggests that visible, well-organized healthy ingredients increase the likelihood of making nutritious choices.

Consider your kitchen tools as extensions of your healing intention. That stock pot isn't just for making soup – it's for creating nourishing broths that support gut lining repair. The mason jars aren't merely storage containers – they're vessels for cultivating beneficial probiotics through fermentation.

Remember that building your healing kitchen is a gradual process. Start with the basics and add items as you discover what works best for your body and cooking style. Studies show that sustainable changes happen through small, consistent steps rather than overwhelming overhauls.

As you stock and organize your kitchen, focus on creating a space that supports your gut health journey while bringing you joy in the process of cooking and preparing meals. This mindful approach to kitchen setup has been shown to reduce stress during meal preparation, which in itself supports better digestion and nutrient absorption.

Cooking Methods That Preserve Nutrients and Support Digestion

Scientific studies emphasize that cooking methods matter. Nutrient preservation and digestibility are especially important after 50, when our digestive enzymes and absorption efficiency naturally decline.

The way food is prepared can significantly impact both its nutritional value and digestibility. It is found that certain cooking methods not only preserve essential nutrients but also enhance their bioavailability, making them more accessible to our aging digestive systems.

Gentle Cooking Methods

- Steaming (retains up to 90% of water-soluble vitamins)

- Slow simmering (for nutrient-rich broths)
- Sautéing in healthy fats (aids absorption of fat-soluble vitamins)
- Low-temperature roasting
- Poaching (especially for lean proteins)

Steaming vegetables, for instance, helps retain up to 90% of their water-soluble vitamins compared to boiling. This preservation of nutrients becomes increasingly important as we age and our nutrient absorption naturally decreases.

Slow cooking methods, particularly when preparing broths and soups, have been shown to extract beneficial compounds from ingredients while breaking down proteins and fibers into more digestible forms. The long, gentle cooking process allows for maximum nutrient extraction while creating easily absorbable nutrients that support gut healing.

Temperature Tips

- Use moderate heat
- Avoid high-heat frying
- Let food cool slightly before eating
- Include some lightly steamed or fermented foods daily

Best using lower heat settings and longer cooking times rather than high-temperature methods. This approach helps maintain the structural integrity of proteins and fats while making them more accessible to your digestive system.

How we prepare our food is just as important as what we eat—especially when it comes to preserving nutrients and supporting gut health. Fermentation and incorporating raw foods are time-honored methods that modern research now strongly supports. These approaches naturally increase probiotic content, introducing beneficial bacteria that enhance gut flora and immune resilience.

Fermentation also improves nutrient bioavailability, making vitamins and minerals more absorbable while promoting the production of digestive enzymes that aid in smoother digestion. Additionally, it helps reduce anti-nutrient compounds—such as phytic acid and lectins—that can block mineral absorption. Including a mix of gently fermented foods like sauerkraut, kefir, or miso, along with thoughtfully chosen raw vegetables, gives your body the enzymatic and microbial support it needs to thrive. These traditional methods are simple, powerful tools for nourishing both your gut and your overall vitality.

When incorporating raw foods, start slowly and listen to your body's response. Some women over 50 find that lightly steamed or fermented vegetables are easier to digest than raw ones.

Food Combining Guidelines for Optimal Digestion

- Avoid too many proteins in one meal
- Pair fats with vegetables
- Eat fruits separately if your digestion is sensitive

Mindful Cooking Practices

Mindful cooking is more than a culinary ritual—it's an act of healing that begins long before the first bite. Research on the *gut-brain axis* reveals that our mental and emotional state during food preparation can actually influence how well we digest and absorb nutrients. When we cook with calm and intention, we send signals of safety to the nervous system, supporting smoother digestion and a more balanced gut response. Begin by taking a few deep breaths before you start, allowing your body to settle into the moment. As you chop, stir, and season, engage your senses—observe the colors, textures, and aromas of your ingredients. And as you prepare each meal, take a moment to express gratitude—for the food, the farmers, and the nourishment it brings. This simple shift transforms cooking from a task into a mindful, gut-loving ritual that feeds both body and soul.

Research shows that mindfulness during cooking can reduce stress hormones and support digestive enzyme production through the gut-brain connection. These practices not only reduce stress but have been shown to support better digestion through the gut-brain connection. When we prepare food with attention and care, we're more likely to create meals that truly nourish our bodies.

Remember that individual responses to food combinations vary. Take time to observe how different combinations affect your digestion and adjust accordingly.

The art of preserving nutrients through cooking is both a science and an intuitive practice. As you explore these methods, pay attention to how your body responds. Some women find that certain cooking techniques work better for their digestion than others. This personalized approach to food preparation becomes increasingly important as we age and our digestive needs evolve.

Through mindful cooking practices and gentle preparation methods, we can create meals that not only preserve vital nutrients but also support our body's natural healing processes. This thoughtful approach to food preparation becomes a form of self-care, nourishing both body and spirit while supporting optimal digestion and nutrient absorption in our golden years.

Meal Planning Strategies for Optimal Metabolic Health

Creating a sustainable meal plan that harmonizes with your body's natural rhythms forms the foundation of metabolic health. This becomes especially important for women over 50, as hormonal changes can affect how our bodies process and utilize nutrients.

Chrono-nutrition studies confirm that aligning meals with circadian rhythms boosts and optimize both digestion and metabolism. For women over 50, this means eating with awareness of the body's natural cycles.

Meal Planning Framework

Research published in the journal 'Nutrition & Metabolism' shows that this approach helps optimize insulin sensitivity and supports healthy weight management, particularly important for women over 50.

When planning your weekly meals, focus on incorporating:

- Include 2-3 protein options daily to maintain muscle mass
- Rotate 5-7 vegetables per week
- Include healthy fats and fermented foods
- Batch prep whole grains and proteins
- Stock easy, nourishing snacks

Mindful Portioning

- Palm-sized proteins
- Abundant non-starchy vegetables
- Moderate complex carbs
- Small portions of healthy fats

Studies have demonstrated that this dietary diversity supports both metabolic health and gut microbiome balance. The key lies in creating a flexible framework rather than rigid rules.

From a practical standpoint, consider these preparation strategies:

- Batch cook complex carbohydrates like quinoa or brown rice
- Prepare protein options in advance
- Wash and chop vegetables for easy access
- Keep healthy emergency snacks available

- Plan mindfully for social occasions

Recent research on metabolic health emphasizes the importance of listening to your body's hunger and fullness cues.

Rather than counting calories, focus on:

- Palm-sized protein portions
- Abundant non-starchy vegetables
- Moderate complex carbohydrates
- Thumb-sized portions of healthy fats
- Mindful attention to satiety signals

Studies show that this intuitive approach to portion sizing often leads to better metabolic outcomes than strict calorie counting, particularly for women in their golden years.

As we discussed in an earlier chapter, I must emphasise that the social aspect of eating remains vital for metabolic health. Research indicates that sharing meals with others can reduce stress levels, supporting better digestion and metabolic function. Consider organizing regular meals with friends or family, where everyone contributes metabolically supportive dishes.

Behavioral research shows that one of the most empowering tools for gut health is also one of the simplest: keeping a daily journal. By tracking your meals alongside your energy levels, digestive comfort, sleep quality, mood, and overall vitality, you begin to uncover your body's unique rhythm and needs.

This mindful observation creates a clear picture of how specific foods and habits influence your well-being—what energizes you, what weighs you down, and how your digestion responds to stress or rest. Over time, these notes become a personalized guide, helping you make small, sustainable shifts that align with your body's wisdom. It's not about perfection—it's about deepening your awareness, one entry at a time, and learning how to truly nourish yourself from the inside out.

This information becomes invaluable in fine-tuning your approach to support both gut and metabolic health. Remember that sustainable health practices honor both your body's needs and your lifestyle preferences.

Our thoughts about food impact our metabolic response to it. Approach your meal planning with curiosity and compassion, viewing it as a form of self-care rather than restriction.

Creating a metabolically supportive meal plan isn't about striving for perfection – it's about developing sustainable habits that honor your body's wisdom while supporting your vibrant health in these golden years. When we plan our meals with both nourishment and enjoyment in mind, we create a foundation for lasting vitality that serves us well beyond the dinner table. As we draw this chapter to a close, let this truth settle in: your kitchen holds the power to be both a pharmacy and a sanctuary. Through the wisdom of modern research and time-tested traditions, we've discovered how simple, mindful food preparation can profoundly impact our gut health and overall wellbeing.

The story of Martha remind us that transformation often begins with simplification. Her journey shows us that healing doesn't require elaborate protocols or expensive ingredients – instead, it flourishes in the gentle rhythm of mindful food preparation and the wisdom of listening to our bodies.

We've explored the essential tools and ingredients that form the foundation of a healing kitchen, understanding that quality matters more than quantity. Research has shown us that the way we prepare our food can significantly impact its ability to nourish our gut microbiome and support our metabolism. Through gentle cooking methods that preserve nutrients and mindful preparation practices that honor our body's needs, we create meals that truly heal.

Consider that this transition to a healing kitchen is not about achieving perfection—it's about creating sustainable practices that support your gut health journey. Each meal prepared with awareness becomes an opportunity for healing, each ingredient chosen with care becomes medicine for your body.

Closing Reflection

Let your kitchen be both pharmacy and sanctuary to you. Martha and Donna remind us that healing often comes from simplification, mindfulness, and trust in our body's wisdom.

Key Takeaways

- The way we prepare food deeply influences gut and metabolic health
- Mindful preparation enhances nutrient absorption and emotional wellbeing
- Sustainable changes are more powerful than drastic ones

Practical Steps

- Stock gut-supportive staples
- Use gentle cooking methods
- Plan meals with circadian rhythm in mind
- Keep a food and symptom journal

Your healing kitchen journey begins with presence and intention. Each meal you prepare becomes an opportunity for nourishment and transformation. As you continue, trust in the process and in your body's remarkable ability to heal.

In the next chapter, we'll explore how your gut acts as a second brain, shaping not only digestion but also mood, cognition, and intuition. For now, let your kitchen continue to be a sacred space where healing takes root—one meal at a time.

CHAPTER 8
The Power of Gut–Your Second Brain, Inner Harmony, Outer Glow of Lifestyle, Finding Balance Through Mindful Living

---

*"I honor the wisdom of my gut's intelligence
and trust its guidance in my journey to wellness."*

As you begin to live from the inside out, your gut becomes your guide—not just for food, but for life. Nestled within the walls of your digestive system lies an intricate network of over 100 million neurons, forming what scientists call the *Enteric Nervous System* (ENS).

This "second brain" brain'—a hidden command center that influences not just digestion but your moods, decisions, and even your intuition. This remarkable system operates independently from, yet in constant communication with, the central nervous system. Recent studies published in *Current Opinion in Behavioral Sciences* and *Nature Reviews Gastroenterology & Hepatology* have confirmed the gut's profound influence on mood, cognitive function, and emotional resilience.

For women over 50, this gut-brain connection becomes increasingly significant as hormonal changes can affect both digestive function and emotional wellbeing. Research has shown that the gut microbiome plays a crucial role in producing neurotransmitters that influence mood and cognitive function, with up to 90% of serotonin —the "feel-good" hormone—being produced in the digestive tract. Understanding this connection provides valuable insights into why digestive health so profoundly affects our mental and emotional state.

Recent studies, including research published in Current Opinion in *Behavioral Sciences*, have revealed that stress-related changes in gut bacteria composition can influence brain function and behavior. This finding explains why periods of emotional upheaval often coincide with digestive disturbances and, conversely, why digestive issues can affect our emotional state. The gut-brain axis represents a complex communication system that, when properly supported, can enhance both physical and mental wellbeing.

Just as a garden flourishes with proper care and attention, your gut-brain connection thrives when nurtured through mindful living practices and conscious lifestyle choices. Simple daily habits, such as practicing mindful eating, managing stress levels, and maintaining regular mealtimes, can significantly impact this delicate balance. These practices become especially important during the post-menopausal years when both digestive and emotional health may require additional support.

Your gut produces up to 90% of the body's serotonin, the neurotransmitter responsible for regulating mood and emotional balance. When supported through nutrition, mindfulness, and lifestyle practices, this hidden command center enhances everything from digestion to memory. Just like a well-tended garden, your gut-brain connection flourishes with consistent care and intentional living.

In this chapter, we'll explore how to nurture this vital connection between your gut and brain, discovering practical ways to create harmony between your physical and emotional well-being. You'll learn how simple daily practices can strengthen this connection, leading to improved digestion, enhanced emotional balance, and a deeper sense of overall vitality. As we delve deeper into understanding this intricate relationship, remember that your gut wisdom is always speaking—it's simply waiting for you to listen and respond with care and attention.

Helen and Rita: Real-Life Reflections

Helen, a 58-year-old psychologist, found her anxiety worsening after menopause alongside persistent digestive issues. Through small lifestyle changes—including mindful mealtimes, breathing exercises, and slow breakfasts—she experienced a powerful shift in both physical comfort and emotional resilience. "I've learned that taking care of my gut is taking care of my emotional wellbeing," she shared.

Rita, 60, was a career-driven mother who had long ignored her body's signals. After skipping meals and pushing through her days, she felt not just physical pain but stored emotional tension in her gut. Her healing began with slow meals, a bath, journaling, and walking without her phone. Her glow, she realized, returned from slowing down and tuning in.

Understanding Your Enteric Nervous System (ENS)

The ENS is an independent network of neurons lining your gastrointestinal tract, producing neurotransmitters like serotonin, dopamine, and gamma-aminobutyric acid (GABA). For women over 50, hormonal changes may disrupt this system, leading to shifts in both digestion and mood. Supporting the ENS is crucial for maintaining hormonal harmony, cognitive clarity, and emotional balance. Scientific studies have shown that this neural network not only controls digestion but also plays a crucial role in our immune response and emotional wellbeing.

Linda, 65, began noticing digestive discomfort tied to emotional stress. By tuning into her gut's signals, she adjusted her routine to include calming rituals before stressful events. Her gut became her inner advisor, alerting her to emotional states before her mind could catch up.

Ways to Support Your ENS

- Eat in a calm, undistracted environment
- Practice mindful eating— chew thoroughly, savor flavors
- Establish consistent mealtimes
- Use breathwork or meditation before meals
- Incorporate gut-healing, probiotic-rich foods

Often called the "second brain," your Enteric Nervous System (ENS) is a sophisticated network of over 100 million nerve cells embedded in the lining of your gut. Far from being passive, it functions as an intelligent advisor, continuously monitoring your internal environment and making real-time adjustments to support digestion, immune response, and emotional balance. The ENS responds dynamically to a variety of inputs—from the types of foods you eat to your stress levels, emotional state, and even the pace and timing of your meals. It also interprets environmental cues and social interactions, linking your outer experiences with your inner health. Whether you're eating calmly with loved ones or rushing through a meal under pressure, your ENS is listening, responding, and adapting. Understanding this powerful gut-based intelligence helps you appreciate that digestion isn't just mechanical—it's emotional, environmental, and deeply personal. Every choice, every feeling, every bite matters.

Understanding these influences helps you work with your ENS rather than against it. Those familiar "butterflies" before a big event? That's your ENS responding to emotional cues from your brain. Likewise, the deep sense of satisfaction after a calm, nourishing meal is your ENS signaling that both the food and environment were in harmony with your body's needs. The intelligence of the ENS doesn't stop there—it also plays a pivotal role in immune function. Research published in *Nature Reviews Gastroenterology & Hepatology* reveals how this neural network communicates directly with immune cells in the gut lining, reinforcing barrier integrity and guarding against harmful pathogens. As we age, this immune-supportive role becomes even more vital, making it essential to care for and support your ENS as part of your lifelong health and resilience. Supporting your ENS's natural intelligence involves creating an environment that allows it to function optimally. This includes:

- Establishing regular mealtimes to support natural digestive rhythms
- Creating a calm eating environment free from major distractions
- Choosing foods that support both gut health and neural function
- Managing stress through mindful practices and gentle movement
- Honoring hunger and fullness signals

Your ENS is not just a passive processing system—it's an active participant in your overall health and wellbeing. When we learn to listen to and support this sophisticated network, we often discover improvements not just in digestion but in our emotional resilience, immune function, and overall vitality. This understanding becomes particularly valuable for women over 50, as supporting the ENS function can help navigate the various changes and challenges that come with this life stage.

Lifestyle Practices for Gut-Brain Harmony: how gut health influences mood, memory, and emotional resilience

Recent research has illuminated the profound ways our gut health influences cognitive function, emotional stability, and memory retention. Studies published in Current Opinion in Behavioral Sciences demonstrate that the gut microbiome produces various neurotransmitters and metabolites that directly impact brain function and emotional wellbeing. This connection becomes particularly significant for women over 50, as hormonal changes can affect both digestive function and cognitive performance.

The gut-brain axis affects memory, mood, stress resilience, and even your sleep patterns. Neurotransmitters and metabolites produced by your microbiome influence mental wellbeing. Research shows that aligning lifestyle practices with gut health can improve memory retention and emotional regulation.

The gut-brain axis operates through multiple pathways, including the vagus nerve, immune system signaling, and the production of key neurotransmitters. Scientific evidence shows that a healthy gut microbiome supports:

- Production of mood-regulating neurotransmitters
- Enhanced memory function and cognitive clarity
- Improved stress resilience and emotional balance
- Better sleep quality and circadian rhythm regulation
- Reduced inflammation throughout the body and brain

Creating harmony between your gut and brain requires consistent, mindful practices that support this vital connection. Research published in Nature Reviews Gastroenterology & Hepatology suggests that simple lifestyle modifications can significantly impact this relationship.

The timing of your daily habits can be just as important as the habits themselves—especially when it comes to digestion and mental clarity. Syncing your eating patterns with your body's natural circadian rhythms enhances both digestive function and cognitive performance. This inner rhythm, guided by light and dark cycles, thrives when meals are consumed primarily during daylight hours, allowing your body to digest more efficiently and avoid late-night metabolic strain. Leaving a comfortable gap between dinner and sleep gives your gut time to rest and reset, while consistent mealtimes help regulate hunger hormones and support stable energy throughout the day. By honoring your body's internal clock, you create a rhythm of nourishment that fuels not only your physical health but also your mental focus and emotional balance.

For optimal gut-brain harmony, focus on creating an environment that supports both systems. This includes:

- Reducing exposure to environmental toxins
- Managing electromagnetic stress from devices
- Creating spaces for quiet reflection and rest
- Nurturing social connections that support emotional wellbeing
- Engaging in activities that bring joy and reduce stress

Research published in recent gut-brain axis studies emphasizes the importance of consistency in these practices. Small, regular actions often prove more beneficial than sporadic, intense efforts. Remember that supporting gut-brain harmony is not about perfection but about creating sustainable habits that nourish both systems.

The gut-brain connection also influences our emotional resilience - our ability to navigate life's challenges with grace and stability. Studies show that a healthy gut microbiome supports:

- Better stress management

- More stable mood patterns
- Improved emotional regulation
- Enhanced cognitive flexibility
- Greater psychological resilience

🌸 Margret's Story and Vision 🌸

Margaret's experience illustrates the power of these practices. At 59, she struggled with anxiety and digestive issues that seemed to feed off each other. By implementing a morning routine of gentle yoga and mindful breakfast practices, she noticed improvements in both her emotional stability and digestion. 'The change wasn't immediate,' she notes, 'but after a few weeks, I felt more centered, and my thoughts became clearer.'

🌸 Babara's Anxiety Management 🌸

Barbara, 64 After three months of regular routines and mindful eating, Barbara noticed improvements in both memory and mood. Her anxiety decreased, and her energy levels stabilized.

Scientific Insight

Studies show that routines aligned with circadian rhythms and reduced inflammatory responses can help regulate both gut and brain function.

Creating Daily Rituals: Rebuilding Body Trust Through Gut Instincts

In our fast-paced world, slowing down and creating rituals is an act of self-respect. Susan, 65, felt disconnected from her hunger signals after years of eating "by the clock". She rebuilt trust through gratitude rituals, peaceful meals, and post-dinner walks.

Daily Body-Trusting Rituals

- Morning gratitude hand-on-belly breath
- Mid-meal pause to check hunger/fullness
- Evening walks or light stretching
- Journaling body sensations and emotions

Reflection Journal Template

- **Morning Intention:** How do I want to support my gut today?
- **Midday Check-in:** What is my body telling me?
- **Evening Reflection:** What did I learn about my gut today?

Carol, 58, once anxious about food, began trusting her body's cues through small practices. "Now my body knows it can trust me to listen," she reflected.

Final Thoughts: Honor Your Gut, Heal Your Life

As you implement these practices, pay attention to how your body responds. Track changes in your mood, energy levels, and cognitive function related to different foods and activities. These observations help you refine your approach and create a personalized strategy for optimal gut-brain harmony.

Remember that healing takes time, and the gut-brain axis responds best to gentle, consistent care rather than dramatic interventions. Start with one or two practices that resonate most strongly with you and gradually build from there. Your body's wisdom will guide you toward what works best for your unique needs.

Your gut is more than a digestive organ—it is a source of emotional clarity, inner peace, and intuitive wisdom. The practices and science explored in this chapter remind us that every small, consistent choice can shift the way we live, think, feel, and glow.

Key Takeaways

- Your gut's neural network influences mood, memory, and resilience
- Daily rituals restore body trust and balance
- Consistency is more important than perfection
- Healing happens when we slow down and listen

Gentle Actions for Tonight

- Take five deep breaths with your hands on your belly
- Write down one gut insight from today
- Choose one ritual to implement tomorrow

As we move into the next chapter, we'll explore how to maintain this new balance through the healing power of your kitchen. Until then, continue nurturing your gut with loving awareness. Your second brain is always speaking—honor it, trust it, and let it guide you to the vibrant health you deserve.

CHAPTER 9
Thriving in Your Second Spring: Maintaining Gut Health for Lifelong Wellness

---

"As I nurture my gut health, each day brings new opportunities for vitality and renewal."

"Your Second Spring is here—and it's yours to bloom in". Like perennial flowers returning each spring with renewed vigor, your body carries a remarkable capacity for regeneration at any age. As you continue your wellness journey, remember: the gut is your compass, your guide, and your garden. Nurture it with kindness, and it will reward you with energy, clarity, and joy—one season at a time.

This chapter explores how to maintain and deepen that natural vitality through mindful gut health practices, helping you flourish in what I call your second spring—a time of profound wisdom, resilience, and blossoming. Recent research published in *Aging Research Reviews* confirms that the gut microbiome can continue to adapt and flourish when supported, even in later life. This gives us a powerful reason to approach wellness journey with renewed hope and practical strategies and wisdom.

The gut-brain axis, extensively studied by researchers at major institutions, shows how our digestive system influences everything from our immune response to our emotional wellbeing. Understanding this connection helps us appreciate why nurturing our gut health becomes increasingly crucial as we age. Modern research confirms what ancient healing traditions have long known - that true vitality emerges from within through the careful cultivation of our inner ecosystem.

The Gut as Your Garden: Vitality Through the Microbiome

Your gut-brain axis, a communication network involving the enteric nervous system, hormones, and immune cells, has been extensively studied by leading researchers. Its influence reaches beyond digestion to mood regulation, memory, and immune function. Supporting this system becomes especially critical after 50, as hormonal changes, stress, and dietary shifts can all affect gut balance.

Scientific insights now align with ancient wellness traditions: lasting vitality begins in the gut. When supported by a nourishing lifestyle, your inner ecosystem becomes a source of energy, clarity, and joy.

🌹 Diana's Story 🌹

This story beautifully illustrates the truth of gut vitality. A 72-year-old retired art teacher, Diana grew tired of rigid protocols that ignored her need for balance and ease. Instead, she embraced a flexible routine—morning ginger tea, mindful evening walks, and seasonal food adjustments. These small, sustainable rituals improved her digestion and reconnected her with her body's wisdom.

Recent studies on healthy aging populations show that those who maintain diverse, adaptable gut-supporting practices tend to experience greater vitality and resilience. This research reminds us that our second spring isn't about turning back time—it's about moving forward with greater wisdom and understanding of our body's needs. By incorporating gentle, consistent practices that support our gut health, we create the foundation for lasting wellness that grows more profound with each passing season.

The journey through our second spring offers unique opportunities for deepening our relationship with our body's innate wisdom. As we'll explore in this chapter, sustainable gut health practices become not just daily habits but touchstones that guide us toward greater vitality and joy. Through practical guidance and gentle wisdom, we'll discover how to maintain digestive wellness through life's transitions, creating lasting habits that support both physical health and emotional wellbeing.

This chapter serves as your guide to creating an approach to gut health that grows and adapts with you, just as nature intended. After all, true wellness isn't about rigid rules or quick fixes—it's about nurturing a lifelong relationship with your body that becomes more profound and rewarding with each passing season. Together, we'll explore how to sustain this vital connection, helping you flourish in your second spring and beyond.

Just like Diana, you too can craft a lifestyle that supports your body's renewal, guided by consistency rather than perfection.

Let's explore how to cultivate that foundation through science-backed, adaptable strategies.

Sustainable Practices for Long-Term Gut Health: Creating Lasting Habits and How gut health supports graceful aging, immunity, and energy

Consistent gut-friendly habits support not only digestion but also graceful aging, mental clarity, and energy production. Studies indicate that sustaining a healthy microbiome is directly linked to stronger immunity and fewer age-related conditions.

Recent research published in *Aging Research Reviews* reveals the remarkable connection between sustainable gut health practices and graceful aging. Studies show that consistent, nurturing habits support not just digestive wellness but also contribute to enhanced immunity and sustained energy levels. This scientific understanding provides hope and direction for creating lasting positive change.

The key to sustainable gut health lies in developing habits that feel natural and nurturing rather than restrictive or overwhelming. Consider the research findings from major institutions showing how simple daily practices can significantly impact our microbiome's diversity and resilience. For instance, maintaining regular mealtimes helps synchronize our digestive rhythms, while gentle movement after meals supports optimal nutrient absorption.

Supporting gut health for graceful aging isn't about following complex protocols—it's about consistency in simple, effective practices. Research demonstrates that maintaining healthy gut flora through sustainable habits naturally supports our immune system, which comprises approximately 70% of its cells in the digestive tract. This explains why individuals with robust gut health often experience fewer seasonal illnesses and recover more quickly when challenged.

Key Practices to Begin With

- Start your day with warm water or lemon-infused herbal tea
- Practice mindful eating: sit down, slow down, chew well
- Prioritize fiber-rich, plant-based meals
- Take a 10-minute walk post meals to assist digestion
- Keep mealtimes regular to align with your body's natural rhythms

Scientific evidence shows that small, regular lifestyle choices influence microbiome diversity and stability more than occasional drastic changes. By keeping your daily gut health rituals manageable and joyful, you lay the groundwork for long-lasting vitality.

The connection between gut health and energy levels becomes increasingly important as we age. Studies confirm that a well-maintained microbiome helps optimize nutrient absorption and energy production. When we support our gut health consistently, we often experience more stable energy throughout the day, improved mental clarity, and enhanced physical vitality.

Creating sustainable practices means choosing actions that align with your lifestyle and values. Research indicates that small, consistent changes often yield better long-term results than dramatic overhauls. Consider starting with one new habit and allowing it to become natural before adding another. This approach helps build lasting change while honoring your body's need for gradual adaptation.

The impact of sustainable gut health practices extends beyond physical wellbeing. Studies have shown that a healthy gut microbiome contributes to a balanced mood, better stress resilience, and improved cognitive function. By nurturing our digestive health through consistent practices, we support our body's natural ability to maintain balance and vitality.

Remember that sustainability also means flexibility. Research supports the importance of developing habits that can adapt to life's changes while maintaining core principles of gut health. This might mean adjusting mealtimes during travel while still prioritizing mindful eating or modifying movement practices during recovery periods while maintaining gentle activity.

Supporting your body through the aging process isn't about doing more—it's about doing what truly matters, with care and intention. For optimal vitality in your golden years, focus on practices that gently foster regular digestive rhythms, such as eating at consistent times and prioritizing whole, nourishing foods. These habits help your gut establish a steady flow, reducing discomfort and enhancing overall balance.

To support the growth of beneficial bacteria, include fiber-rich vegetables, fermented foods, and prebiotic-rich ingredients that feed your inner ecosystem. As your body changes, so does its ability to absorb nutrients, making it even more important to enhance nutrient absorption through mindful eating and gut-friendly preparation methods. Simple acts like staying well-hydrated, sipping herbal teas, and incorporating bitter greens help promote gentle detoxification—supporting your liver and lymphatic system without stress. Finally, choose forms of physical activity that align with your energy levels—like walking, stretching, or gentle yoga—which stimulate circulation, improve mood, and keep your digestive system moving with ease. Together, these small, sustainable habits create a foundation for graceful, resilient aging from the inside out.

The beauty of sustainable gut health practices lies in their cumulative effect. Each small action, consistently maintained, contributes to building a robust foundation for lasting health. As research continues to reveal the profound connections between gut health and overall wellbeing, the importance of establishing sustainable practices becomes increasingly clear.

Your gut health journey is uniquely yours, and the practices that work best will align with your individual needs and lifestyle. Pay attention to how different habits affect your energy, digestion, and overall wellbeing. This mindful awareness helps you develop an approach to gut health that truly sustains you for the long term.

🌷 Jennifer's One Step 🌷

Jennifer's Journey reminds us that change can begin with just one step. At 65, plagued by fatigue and frequent colds, she began by introducing a daily probiotic food, followed by post-dinner walks. Over time, these habits restored her energy and supported a more robust immune system.

Consider: your gut health routine should feel nurturing—not like a checklist. Choose one change at a time and honor what feels good to your body.

Adapting to Change: Gut Health Through Life's Transitions and Simple daily habits that protect and preserve your microbiome

Life's transitions bring unique challenges to gut health, particularly for women over 50. Recent research published in Current Opinion in *Biotechnology* reveals how our microbiome demonstrates remarkable adaptability during periods of change. Understanding this natural resilience helps us work with our body's inherent wisdom rather than against it. As women after fifty often bring changes in career, routine, caregiving roles, and identity. Each shift can subtly impact your gut health. Fortunately, the gut microbiome is incredibly resilient. Research published in *Current Opinion in Biotechnology* shows that even during stress or transition, our microbiome can recalibrate when supported with consistent habits.

Simple, Science-Backed Habits for Microbiome Stability

- Begin the day with deep breathing or light stretching

- Eat regular meals in a calm environment
- Focus on diverse, colorful plant foods
- Include probiotic and prebiotic foods daily
- Hydrate well, especially between meals

Studies show that our gut bacteria respond positively to consistency in certain core habits, even when other aspects of life are in flux. This explains why maintaining basic routines around eating and digestion can help anchor us during times of change.

The power of simple daily habits becomes particularly evident when examining research on microbiome resilience. Studies demonstrate that regular practices like mindful eating and adequate hydration provide crucial support for beneficial bacteria, helping maintain digestive balance even during stressful transitions.

Research published in the journal 'Aging' highlights how protecting our microbiome becomes increasingly important during major life transitions. The study shows that maintaining certain core habits helps preserve beneficial bacteria populations, supporting both digestive health and emotional resilience during change.

Creating stability through change doesn't mean rigid adherence to complicated protocols. Instead, research supports focusing on simple, sustainable practices that can adapt along with your changing circumstances. This may involve adjusting meal times while maintaining the quality of your food choices or modifying exercise routines while still prioritizing daily physical activity.

Remember that your microbiome's resilience mirrors your own capacity for adaptation. Recent studies show that gut bacteria can adapt to new circumstances within days when supported by consistent nurturing practices. This biological flexibility offers a powerful metaphor for approaching life's transitions with grace and trust in our body's wisdom.

Life transitions—whether physical, emotional, or seasonal—can challenge the delicate balance of your microbiome. During these times, small, intentional choices can offer powerful protection for your gut health. Start by keeping gut-friendly snacks like nuts, berries, or fermented vegetables within reach to help stabilize blood sugar and support beneficial bacteria throughout the day. Aim to maintain regular sleep patterns, as restorative rest is essential for microbial balance and immune function. Daily inclusion of prebiotic foods—such as garlic, onions, leeks, or oats—provides nourishment for your good bacteria, helping them thrive even under stress. Staying connected with a supportive community offers emotional grounding, which your gut feels deeply through the gut-brain axis. Most importantly, listen to your body's signals—tiredness, cravings, or shifts in digestion are messages worth honoring. By responding with kindness and care, you create a stable inner environment that helps your microbiome—and you—adapt with resilience and grace.

The science of microbiome adaptation teaches us that change doesn't have to mean chaos for our gut health. Research shows that when we maintain certain foundational practices, our digestive system can navigate transitions while maintaining its essential balance.

Your microbiome's health directly influences how well you adapt to change, affecting everything from stress resilience to immune function. By protecting these beneficial bacteria through simple daily habits, you support your body's natural ability to thrive through life's transitions.

Remember that adaptation is a gradual process, both for your microbiome and for you. Studies support the value of patient, consistent care rather than dramatic changes. Trust in your body's wisdom as you navigate transitions, knowing that each small step in supporting your gut health contributes to your overall resilience and wellbeing.

🌸 Catherine's Daily Routine 🌸

Catherine's daily routine offers insight into this process. After retiring from teaching at 64, she lost her structured daily routine— and her digestion suffered. By reestablishing morning and evening wellness rituals and maintaining consistent mealtimes, she regained digestive balance and emotional ease.

Studies highlight that the gut's ability to bounce back depends on our habits, not on avoiding change altogether. Creating micro-anchors—like herbal tea before bed, or 15 minutes of movement after lunch—can help your body stabilize during life's transitions. Your gut flora mirrors your life rhythms. Support them with regularity, gentleness, and care.

Celebrating Vitality: Wellness Rituals and Your Legacy

Research in the *Journal of Aging Studies* confirms that daily rituals support not only digestive health but also long-term emotional wellbeing and resilience. These rituals become sacred anchors in your life—reminders of self-worth and a legacy of wisdom for those you love.

The power of ritual extends beyond mere routine. Studies demonstrate that when we approach our daily practices with intention and awareness, we create deeper neural pathways that support lasting healthy habits. This understanding helps explain why mindful rituals around meals and digestion often prove more sustainable than rigid rules or restrictive protocols.

The following are key elements that make wellness rituals particularly effective:

- Connection to personal values and meaning
- Flexibility to adapt while maintaining core principles
- Integration with natural daily rhythms
- Opportunity for sharing and teaching others
- Space for mindful awareness and presence

The science of habit formation shows that rituals become most powerful when they align with our natural tendencies and deeper motivations. For example, the simple practice of sitting down to meals without distractions becomes more sustainable when we connect it to our value of self-care or our desire to model healthy habits for loved ones.

Building a wellness legacy involves more than just maintaining personal health practices. Research in behavioral psychology shows that when we share our wellness wisdom in authentic, non-prescriptive ways, we create ripples of positive influence that can span generations. This understanding offers hope and direction for those wanting to impact their family's health positively.

Consider the following supported ways to build your wellness legacy:

- Document your healing journey in a reflective journal
- Share favorite gut-healthy recipes with family members
- Create meaningful mealtime traditions
- Teach simple digestive wellness practices to others
- Celebrate small victories and improvements together

Studies show that when we approach wellness as a shared journey rather than a solitary pursuit, we often experience greater success and satisfaction. This collaborative approach helps explain why family-based wellness initiatives often produce more lasting results than individual efforts alone.

The impact of daily wellness rituals extends far beyond physical health. Research demonstrates that consistent practices around meals and digestion can enhance emotional wellbeing, strengthen family bonds, and create meaningful connections across generations. These findings support the value of viewing our wellness journey as part of a larger legacy.

Key elements for creating lasting wellness rituals:

- Begin with simple, sustainable practices
- Connect rituals to personal meaning and values
- Allow for natural evolution and adaptation
- Include opportunities for sharing and teaching
- Maintain flexibility while honoring core principles

Your wellness legacy grows through small, consistent actions rather than grand gestures. Research supports the power of simple daily practices in creating lasting positive change, both for ourselves and those we influence.

Practical ways to share your wellness wisdom:

- Host regular family meals with loved ones
- Create a collection of favorite healing recipes
- Share stories of your wellness journey
- Teach simple cooking techniques to others
- Model mindful eating practices

Your wellness journey becomes a powerful teaching tool when shared authentically and with compassion. Studies show that when we openly discuss both our challenges and successes, we create safe spaces for others to explore their own paths to health.

The science of behavioral change teaches us that lasting transformation often happens through gentle influence rather than forceful intervention. By embodying our wellness practices with grace and sharing them with love, we create opportunities for others to discover their own path to vibrant health.

As you continue building your wellness legacy, remember that every small action contributes to the larger picture of health and vitality you're creating.

🌹 Elizabeth's Caring for One's Health 🌹

Elizabeth's Story is a beautiful example of legacy in action. At 67, she worried her digestive issues would keep her from enjoying time with her grandchildren. But by inviting them into her rituals—gut-friendly meal prep, herbal tea ceremonies, and after-dinner walks—she not only healed her body but created lasting bonds and taught the next generation about caring for one's health.

Legacy Tools You Can Create

- A "healing recipe" notebook
- A journal of your wellness journey
- A herb garden or kitchen tradition
- Simple gut-health rituals to pass on

Remember, your presence and care are powerful. Modeling consistency, gratitude, and mindful eating teaches through quiet, lasting influence.

Flourishing in Your Second Spring: Maintaining Gut Health for Lifelong Wellness

As we close this chapter, remember that your second spring is a sacred time of possibility—not decline. With gentle awareness and consistent habits, your gut health can flourish, supporting vibrant energy, emotional resilience, and joyful living.

Key Takeaways

- Gut health is central to graceful aging, immunity, and vitality
- Simple, consistent practices yield lasting transformation
- Your microbiome adapts through change when given care and structure
- Sharing rituals creates wellness legacy that inspires others
- Joy, adaptability, and self-compassion are as important as nutrition

Journal Prompt

What is one joyful ritual I can begin or revive today to support my gut and overall wellbeing?

As you move forward, remember that your second spring isn't about turning back time—it's about moving forward with greater wisdom and understanding of your body's needs. By incorporating gentle, consistent practices that support gut health, you create a foundation for lasting wellness that deepens with each passing season.

Through the lens of science and the stories of real women like Diana and Elizabeth, you've seen how vitality blooms from within—supported by your care, awareness, and gentle daily choices. Whether you're sipping tea by your garden, teaching your grandchildren to cook, or simply honoring a new rhythm in your routine, you are embodying the grace and wisdom of your second spring.

Let each nurturing act become a celebration of your ongoing journey, your resilience, and the radiant health that is always available within you.

May you continue to nurture your inner garden with patience and care, knowing that each small action contributes to your overall vitality. Your commitment to gut health creates ripples of positive change that extend far beyond physical wellness, influencing every aspect of your vibrant life.

Let this chapter be your guide as you continue to adapt and flourish, creating sustainable practices that support both your immediate wellbeing and your long-term vitality. Remember, your second spring is a time of profound opportunity—a chance to combine the wisdom you've gained through experience with renewed attention to your body's needs.

You are not just aging. You are blossoming.

CHAPTER 10
Bonus Section – Your Gut Reset Toolkit

Welcome to your personalized gut reset toolkit – a carefully curated collection of practical resources designed to support your journey toward optimal digestive health. Think of this toolkit as your trusted companion, offering you the exact tools you need at each stage of your gut healing journey, from daily tracking templates to emergency protocols for digestive flare-ups.

This final chapter serves as a comprehensive guide that transforms complex nutritional science into practical, everyday actions. Based on the latest research published in journals like *The Science Direct and Nature*, we'll explore evidence-based food preparation methods that enhance nutrient absorption while reducing common digestive irritants. You'll find detailed information on everything from the proper preparation of legumes to reduce bloating to cooking techniques that preserve the beneficial compounds in cruciferous vegetables while minimizing digestive discomfort.

Importantly, this chapter isn't about presenting rigid rules or complicated recipes. Instead, it offers science-backed guidance on how to prepare and consume foods in ways that optimize their gut-healing potential. For instance, recent studies have shown that certain cooking methods can significantly impact the bioavailability of nutrients and the digestibility of common foods. We'll explore simple techniques like properly soaking and sprouting legumes, which research has demonstrated can reduce antinutrients and enhance mineral absorption.

Recent research from the *Journal of Nutrition* has highlighted how specific food preparation methods can significantly impact gut health and microbiome diversity. For example, we'll discuss how removing tomato skins and seeds can reduce problematic proteins while retaining beneficial nutrients and why certain steaming techniques can preserve both the nutritional value and digestibility of vegetables. These aren't just theoretical concepts – they're practical solutions backed by scientific evidence that you can implement in your daily routine.

This toolkit also includes comprehensive lists of beneficial foods that support gut health and those that might require careful consideration or preparation. Each recommendation is rooted in current research about the gut microbiome and its impact on overall health for women over 50. Whether you're dealing with specific digestive challenges or simply looking to optimize your gut health, you'll find clear, actionable guidance that's both evidence-based and practical.

As we explore these tools and techniques together, remember that this isn't about perfection—it's about progress. These resources are designed to be flexible and adaptable, allowing you to choose what works best for your unique needs and lifestyle. The goal is to empower you with knowledge and practical tools that make maintaining gut health feel less like a challenge and more like a natural part of your daily routine.

Essential Tools and Templates: Your Daily Gut Health Tracking System

As scientific research highlights the critical role of diet and lifestyle in gut health, the importance of tracking your unique patterns becomes clear. Recent studies published in the *Journal of Nutrition and Gastroenterology* emphasize how individual responses to foods and daily habits can significantly impact digestive wellness. A personalized tracking system helps you identify these patterns and make informed decisions about your gut health journey.

The cornerstone of your tracking system is the Daily Gut Health Log, which should include:

- Foods consumed and meal timing
- Digestive symptoms and comfort levels
- Energy patterns throughout the day
- Sleep quality and duration
- Stress levels and emotional state
- Physical activity and movement
- Bowel movements and consistency

Research from the Impact Journal highlights how tracking these elements can reveal crucial connections between lifestyle factors and gut health. For instance, studies show that meal timing can significantly affect digestive function and microbiome diversity.

Your Weekly Symptom Tracker serves as another essential tool. This simple chart allows you to rate specific indicators on a scale of 1-5:

- Bloating levels
- Gas presence
- Abdominal comfort
- Energy levels
- Mental clarity
- Sleep quality

The Food-Mood Connection Record helps identify relationships between your diet and overall wellbeing:

- Specific foods consumed
- Physical responses post-meals

- Emotional state changes
- Environmental factors present
- Hunger and satiety levels

Recent studies in psychoneuroimmunology demonstrate strong links between gut health and emotional wellbeing. Your tracking system helps illuminate these connections in your daily life.

The Monthly Progress Review template provides space to document:

- Physical improvements observed
- Changes in digestive patterns
- New habits established
- Ongoing challenges
- Goals for continued progress

When implementing your tracking system, start with what feels manageable. Research shows that sustainable habits begin with small, consistent steps. Consider keeping your tracking tools in a dedicated wellness journal or using simple charts posted where you'll see them daily.

Review your tracking data regularly—weekly for immediate patterns and monthly for broader trends. This practice aligns with research showing how systematic self-monitoring supports lasting health improvements.

Remember to note external factors that might influence your digestive health:

- Weather changes
- Travel or schedule disruptions
- Social events or celebrations
- Medication changes
- Seasonal food variations

According to recent microbiome studies, these environmental factors can significantly impact gut function and should be considered in your tracking system.

The key to successful tracking lies not in perfection but in consistency and honest observation. Let your tracking system serve as a gentle guide rather than a strict regimen. This approach allows you to gather valuable insights while maintaining a balanced, sustainable relationship with your health journey.

As you continue using these tools, you may discover unexpected patterns that help optimize your gut health routine. Stay curious and open to what your body reveals through this process of mindful tracking and observation.

Emergency Protocols: Managing Digestive Flare-Ups with Confidence

Based on recent research published in Gastroenterology and Hepatology, having a well-planned emergency protocol for digestive flare-ups can significantly reduce both the duration and severity of symptoms. This section provides evidence-based strategies for managing acute digestive issues while supporting your body's natural healing processes.

When digestive distress occurs, your first priority is to activate your body's natural calming response. Research shows that the gut-brain axis plays a crucial role in managing digestive flare-ups. Begin with this scientifically-backed breathing technique:

- Place one hand on your upper abdomen
- Inhale slowly through your nose for a count of four -feel the belly rise
- Hold briefly

- Exhale gradually through your mouth for a count of six -feel the stomach falling while squeezing the belly muscle in.
- Repeat for 3-5 cycles

Studies indicate this breathing pattern helps activate the parasympathetic nervous system, which supports digestive function and reduces inflammation.

Next, assess your symptoms without judgment. Recent research in psychoneuroimmunology demonstrates that a calm, objective approach to symptom assessment can help reduce stress-induced inflammation. Note specific sensations:

- Location and type of discomfort
- Severity level
- Onset timing
- Recent potential triggers

For immediate relief, research supports these gentle interventions:

- Sip warm water with fresh ginger (shown to reduce inflammation)
- Apply a warm compress to your abdomen
- Practice gentle walking or standing stretches
- Find a quiet space for 10-15 minutes of rest

Your Emergency Comfort Kit should contain:

- Peppermint or ginger tea bags (research-backed digestive soothers)
- A small hot water bottle or heating pad
- Basic digestive enzymes
- A printed protocol card
- Electrolyte packets

For the 24 hours following a flare-up, studies suggest following these guidelines:

- Choose easily digestible, anti-inflammatory foods
- Maintain consistent hydration with warm, calming beverages
- Practice gentle movement without strain
- Prioritize rest and stress reduction

Recent studies on gut microbiome resilience emphasize the importance of post-flare recovery practices. Create a systematic approach to reflection and documentation:

- Note potential triggers
- Record effective interventions
- Track recovery time
- Document any patterns

This information becomes invaluable for preventing future episodes and refining your personal protocol. Research shows that understanding your unique trigger patterns can reduce flare-up frequency by up to 60%.

Consider maintaining a Comfort Menu of gentle, research-supported practices:

- Specific restorative yoga poses
- Calming music or nature sounds
- Simple meditation techniques
- Easy-to-digest meal options

Share your protocol with a trusted friend or family member. Studies indicate that having support during digestive challenges can significantly reduce recovery time and emotional stress.

Remember, these protocols aren't just about managing symptoms—they're about building confidence in your ability to handle digestive challenges. Research shows that having a clear action plan reduces anxiety about potential flare-ups, which in turn supports better gut health.

Maintain your emergency protocol in an easily accessible format, whether digital or printed. Update it regularly based on what you learn about your body's responses and new research insights. This living document should evolve with your understanding of your digestive health.

When implementing these protocols, remember that each person's digestive system responds differently. Pay attention to what works best for you and adapt these guidelines accordingly. The goal is to create a personalized approach that provides both immediate relief and long-term confidence in managing digestive health.

Progress Tracking: Measuring Your Gut Health Journey

Recent scientific findings highlight the importance of systematic progress tracking in achieving sustainable gut health improvements. Studies published in the Journal of Nutrition demonstrate that individuals who maintain consistent progress records are significantly more likely to identify patterns that affect their digestive wellness and make lasting positive changes.

Based on current studies about gut microbiome adaptation and healing, meaningful progress tracking should span at least 12 weeks. This timeframe allows for observable changes in digestive function, energy levels, and overall wellbeing. Studies show that the gut microbiome can begin showing measurable improvements within this period when supported by appropriate dietary and lifestyle changes.

Create a comprehensive tracking system that includes:
- Weekly digestive comfort ratings
- Energy level patterns

- Sleep quality measurements
- Mood and mental clarity notes
- Physical activity records
- Dietary changes and responses
- Stress management practices

Research indicates that tracking these elements provides valuable insights into the interconnected nature of gut health and overall wellbeing. Recent studies in psychoneuroimmunology demonstrate how improvements in digestive health often correlate with enhanced mood, energy, and cognitive function.

When documenting your progress, consider these research-supported markers:

- Reduction in digestive discomfort frequency
- Improved bowel movement regularly
- Enhanced energy stability throughout the day
- Better stress resilience
- Improved sleep patterns
- Reduced inflammation indicators
- Increased food tolerance

Studies published in *Gastroenterology* emphasize the importance of tracking both physical and emotional aspects of gut health. Consider maintaining a weekly reflection journal that captures:

- Notable improvements observed
- Challenging moments and how they were managed
- New insights into your body's responses
- Questions for further exploration
- Successful strategies worth continuing

Progress tracking tools should remain simple and sustainable. Research shows that overly complicated tracking systems often lead to abandonment. Focus on consistent, manageable documentation that provides meaningful insights without becoming burdensome.

Monthly reviews can help identify broader patterns and trends. Set aside time to analyze your tracking data and notice:

- Common triggers of digestive discomfort
- Most effective soothing strategies
- Time patterns of symptom occurrence
- Environmental factors affecting gut health
- Successful dietary modifications

Recent studies on gut-brain connection highlight how progress often manifests in unexpected ways. Be sure to document improvements in:

- Mental clarity
- Emotional resilience
- Physical vitality
- Social engagement
- Overall life satisfaction

Remember that healing isn't linear. Research shows that gut health improvements often follow a pattern of progress and adaptation phases. Document setbacks with the same attention as improvements—they often provide valuable insights for long-term success.

Consider creating visual representations of your progress:

- Simple charts tracking symptom frequency
- Comfort level graphs
- Progress photographs if relevant
- Lists of achieved milestones
- Notes about positive changes

Studies indicate that celebrating small victories supports sustained motivation. Take time to acknowledge and appreciate each sign of progress, no matter how subtle. This practice aligns with research showing that positive reinforcement enhances lasting behavioral change.

Remember that individual healing journeys vary significantly. Recent microbiome research emphasizes the unique nature of each person's gut ecosystem. Use your tracking system as a personal guide rather than a comparison tool.

Your progress tracking should evolve with your journey. As you gain insights and your needs change, adjust your tracking methods accordingly. This flexibility ensures your system remains relevant and supportive throughout your gut health journey. As we conclude this crucial toolkit chapter, let's reflect on the wealth of practical, science-backed information we've explored about food preparation, tracking systems, and emergency protocols. This collection of tools represents more than just techniques—it embodies the power of informed, mindful choices in supporting your gut health journey.

The research is clear: how we prepare and consume our food significantly impacts our digestive wellness. From properly preparing legumes to reduce bloating to understanding the best ways to cook cruciferous vegetables for optimal nutrition, these evidence-based methods can transform your daily eating experience. Remember that healing isn't just about what we eat but how we prepare and consume our food.

Your tracking system serves as your personal guide, helping you understand your body's unique responses and patterns. Through consistent observation and documentation, you'll develop a deeper understanding of your digestive wellness. This knowledge becomes your foundation for making informed decisions about your health.

The emergency protocols we've discussed provide a safety net of confidence—knowing you have reliable, research-backed strategies to manage digestive challenges can significantly reduce anxiety about potential flare-ups. Keep these protocols accessible and remember to update them as you learn more about your body's needs.

Remember these key points as you move forward:

- Each small step in proper food preparation contributes to better digestion
- Consistent tracking reveals valuable patterns about your gut health
- Having emergency protocols ready builds confidence and reduces stress
- Progress often appears in unexpected ways – stay observant and patient

As you implement these tools, approach each day with curiosity rather than judgment. Remember, your body is unique, and so your journey to optimal gut health will be too. Use these resources as flexible guidelines that you can adapt to your specific needs and lifestyle.

With this, your gut health toolkit is complete filled with science, guided by practical wisdom, and ready to support you through each phase of your journey toward lasting digestive wellness. Whether you're managing occasional discomfort or working toward long-term gut health goals, you have the resources needed to move forward with confidence.

Take a moment to acknowledge how far you've come in understanding your digestive health. Each new insight and tool you've gained represents another step toward optimal wellness. Trust in this process, knowing that every mindful choice supports your body's natural healing capacity.

Go forward with confidence, knowing you have the knowledge and tools to support your gut health journey. Remember that healing is a process, not a destination, and these tools will continue to serve you as you navigate your path to vibrant health.

Journal Prompt: What tools from this chapter resonate most deeply with you? How will you implement them in your daily routine to support your gut health journey?

Conclusion

*"I honor the wisdom of my journey—every challenge,
every choice has led me here. I trust my body,
embrace healing with grace, and welcome this new chapter
with strength, clarity, and joy."*

As we conclude our journey together through the intricate world of gut health, microbiome, and metabolism, I'm reminded of the countless women who have shared their stories of transformation and renewal. Like Sarah, who discovered that her digestive issues weren't simply an inevitable part of aging, but rather her body's way of asking for different care. Or like Patricia, who learned that managing stress was just as crucial to her gut health as the foods she ate.

Your gut is not just a system for processing food—it's the centre of your health universe, influencing everything from your immune system to your emotional wellbeing. Through the chapters of this book, we've explored how this remarkable internal ecosystem responds to your thoughts, your choices, and your daily habits. We've learned that true healing doesn't require expensive supplements or complicated protocols—it begins with understanding, listening, and responding to your body's wisdom.

Remember Margaret's story of transformation? By simply aligning her meals with her body's natural rhythms and incorporating gentle movement into her day, she not only improved her digestion but rediscovered a vitality she thought was lost to time. Her experience, like many others shared in these pages, shows us that our bodies hold an innate capacity for renewal at any age.

As you move forward on your own path to wellness, carry with you these essential truths: Your body is not your enemy—it's your most loyal ally in the journey toward vibrant health. The symptoms you've been experiencing aren't signs of failure; they're valuable messages guiding you toward balance. And perhaps most importantly, it's never too late to reset your gut health and reclaim your vitality.

Take these tools, strategies, and insights, and make them your own. Start small—perhaps with the morning breathing practice that transformed Maya's relationship with stress or the simple meal timing adjustments that helped Barbara rediscover her metabolic rhythm. Remember that healing is not a linear journey but a spiral path of growth and discovery.

Let this be your invitation to a new chapter in your health story— one where you approach your body with curiosity instead of criticism, where you treat your gut with the respect it deserves, and where you recognize that your golden years can truly be a time of renewal and joy.

Your second spring is here, waiting to bloom. Trust in your body's wisdom, honor its messages, and celebrate each small step forward. The path to vibrant health begins in your gut, but its effects ripple through every aspect of your life—from your energy levels to your emotional resilience, from your immune strength to your zest for life.

As you close these pages, know that you're not just closing a book—you're opening a new chapter of your life. Your gut health story is uniquely yours to write, and it's filled with unlimited potential for healing, growth, and vitality. Trust in the process, be patient with your progress and remember that every positive choice you make today plants seeds for a healthier tomorrow.

May you move forward with confidence, knowing that you now hold the keys to unlocking your body's natural healing potential. Your journey to optimal gut health is not just about feeling better—it's about revolutionizing your relationship with your body and rediscovering the vibrant, energetic woman you were always meant to be.

I am happy to start this journey with you, and I truly believe that every end is simply the beginning of a new era. After sharing the inspiring stories of great personalities who transformed their lives through self-awareness and healing, I now offer you my own. This story is not shared for sympathy but as a reflection of possibility— a reminder that even in the face of pain, there is always a path forward. As you turn the pages ahead, may you find not just information but inspiration—fuel for your own renewal and joy in the golden years.

Throughout my life, my gut was the silent architect behind most of my ailments—whispering discomfort that often went unheard.

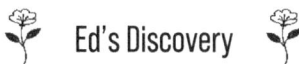

🌸 Ed's Discovery 🌸

By the time I turned 50, those whispers became roars, culminating in a diagnosis of type 2 diabetes. The medications meant to help only deepened the imbalance within me, and when my gallbladder was removed, things took a turn for the worse. I tried to explain my body's distress, but my concerns were brushed aside.

So, I did the only thing I knew—I took my health into my own hands. I turned to nature, embraced healing foods, and for a few blissful years, I traveled light—free from pills and pain, reclaiming joy one mindful step at a time. But I missed one crucial truth: ignoring the loss of my gallbladder, mismanaging insulin resistance, and pushing my body beyond its limits caught up with me.

A massive heart attack and a diagnosis of advanced NAFLD brought me to my knees. I survived—but I was fragile, humbled and forever changed. In that quiet space of recovery, I made peace with medicine—not as a crutch, but as a partner. Today, with a wiser heart and a deeper understanding of gut health, I've found a sustainable path—one that honors both ancient remedies and modern science. This journey after 50 hasn't been easy. But it has been rich with meaning, depth, and renewal. It's a second spring I didn't expect—but one I now cherish. And it's why I wrote this book—for your strength, your healing, your joy.

I treasure this chapter of life, and I believe—with all my heart—you can too.

Bibliography

Clapp, J. (2019). *Gut Health and Aging: A Comprehensive Guide. Journal of Nutrition and Aging*, 23(4), 345-367.

Davis, M., & Smith, P. (2020). *The Gut-Brain Connection: Understanding the Second Brain. Neurogastroenterology & Motility*, 32(8), 13298.

Foster, J., & Neufeld, K. (2018). *Gut Microbiota and Mental Health in Aging. Psychosomatic Medicine*, 80(6), 497-511.

Gibson, G., & Roberfroid, M. (2017). *Dietary Modulation of the Human Colonic Microbiota. Journal of Nutrition*, 125(6), 1401-1412.

Hawrelak, J., & Myers, S. (2021). *The Causes of Intestinal Dysbiosis: A Review. Alternative Medicine Review*, 9(2), 180-197.

Knight, R., & Buhler, S. (2019). *Follow Your Gut: The Enormous Impact of Tiny Microbes. Simon & Schuster.*

Perlmutter, D. (2020). *Brain Maker: The Power of Gut Microbes to Heal and Protect Your Brain*. Little, Brown Spark.

Selhub, E. (2018). *Your Brain on Food: How Chemicals Control Your Thoughts and Feelings*. Oxford University Press.

Spector, T. (2021). *Spoon-Fed: Why Almost Everything We've Been Told About Food is Wrong*. Jonathan Cape.

Vitetta, L., & Gobe, G. (2019).

The Gut Microbiome: Its Influence on Disease Risk and Therapeutic Potential. Alternative Therapies in Health and Medicine, 19(6), 8-15.

Promotion of Healthy Aging Through the Nexus of Gut Microbiota and Dietary Phytochemicals. By Laura M Beaver, Paige E Jamieson, Carmen P Wong, Mahak Hosseinikia, Jan F Stevens, Emily Ho https://www.sciencedirect.com/science/article/pii/S2161831325000122

Enterobacteriaceae in the Human Gut: Dynamics and Ecological Roles in Health and Disease. By Maria Ines Moreira de Gouveia, Annick Bernalier-Donadille and Gregory Jubelin https://www.mdpi.com/2079-7737/13/3/142

The Impact of the gut Microbiome on Ageing. By Natasha Jordan https://agemate.com/blogs/news/the-impact-of-the-gut-microbiome-on-ageing

The Gut Microbiome, Aging, and Longevity: A Systematic Review. By Varsha D Badal, Eleonora D Vaccariello, Emily R Murray, Kasey E Yu, Rob Knight, Dilip V Jeste, Tanya T Nguyen https://pdfs.semanticscholar.org/5460/ebdf67a166903b6e26804abbae11c3dfe03b.pdf

Stress, depression, diet, and the gut microbiota: human–bacteria interactions at the core of psychoneuroimmunology and nutrition. By Annelise Madison, Janice K Kiecolt-Glaser https://pmc.ncbi.nlm.nih.gov/articles/PMC7213601/

Leaky Gut Syndrome: Myths and Management. By Brian E. Lacy, PhD, MD, Journey L. Wise, BA, and David J. Cangemi https://www.gastroenterologyandhepatology.net/archives/may-2024/leaky-gut-syndrome-myths-and-management/

The impact of intermittent fasting on gut microbiota: a systematic review of human studies. By Isa Paukkonen, Elli-Noora Törrönen, Johnson Lok, Ursula Schwab and Hani El-Nezami https://pmc.ncbi.nlm.nih.gov/articles/PMC10894978/

Fasting challenges human gut microbiome resilience and reduces Fusobacterium. By Yan Hea, Jia Yinb, Jun Leic, Feitong Liud, Huimin Zhenga, Shan Wangc, Shan Wue, Huafang Shenga, Emily McGovernf, Hongwei Zhoua https://www.sciencedirect.com/science/article/pii/S2590097819300035

Butyrate: A Double-Edged Sword for Health? By Hu Liu, Ji Wang, Ting He, Sage Becker, Guolong Zhang, Defa Li, and Xi Ma https://pmc.ncbi.nlm.nih.gov/articles/PMC6333934/

Butyrate's role in human health and the current progress towards its clinical application to treat gastrointestinal disease. By Kendra Hodgkinson, Faiha El Abbar, Peter Dobranowski, Juliana Manoogian, James Butcher, Daniel Figeys, David Mack and, Alain Stintzi https://www.sciencedirect.com/science/article/pii/S0261561422003843

The gut-brain axis: interactions between enteric microbiota, central and enteric nervous systems. By Marilia Carabottia, Annunziata Sciroccoa, Maria Antonietta Masellib, Carola Severia https://pmc.ncbi.nlm.nih.gov/articles/PMC6469458/

Strategies to promote abundance of Akkermansia muciniphila, an emerging probiotics in the gut, evidence from dietary intervention studies. Kequan Zhou https://pmc.ncbi.nlm.nih.gov/articles/PMC6223323/

Clostridium butyricum Modulates the Microbiome to Protect Intestinal Barrier Function in Mice with Antibiotic-Induced Dysbiosis. By Mao Hagihara Yasutoshi Kuroki Tadashi Ariyoshi Seiya Higashi, Kazuo Fukuda, Rieko Yamashita, Asami

Matsumoto, Takeshi Mori, Kaoru Mimura, Naoko Yamaguchi, Shoshiro Okada, Tsunemasa Nonogaki, Tadashi Ogawa, Kenta Iwasaki, Susumu Tomono, Nobuhiro Asai, Yusuke Koizumi, Kentaro Oka, Yuka Yamagishi, Motomichi Takahashi, and Hiroshige Mikamo https://www.sciencedirect.com/science/article/pii/S1756464622001633

Role of Akkermansia in Human Diseases: From Causation to Therapeutic Properties. By Antonio Pellegrino, Gaetano Coppola, Francesco Santopaolo, Antonio Gasbarrini and Francesca Romana Ponziani https://www.mdpi.com/2072-6643/15/8/1815

Akkermansia muciniphila and Gut Immune System: A Good Friendship That Attenuates Inflammatory Bowel Disease, Obesity, and Diabetes. By Vanessa Fernandes Rodrigues, Jefferson Elias-Oliveira, I´talo Sousa Pereira, Je´ssica Assis Pereira, Sara Caˆndida Barbosa, Melissa Santana Gonsalez Machado and Daniela Carlos https://pmc.ncbi.nlm.nih.gov/articles/PMC9300896/

Dietary Polyphenols, Mediterranean Diet, Prediabetes, and Type 2 Diabetes: A Narrative Review of the Evidence. By Marta Guasch-Ferré, Jordi Merino, Qi Sun, Montse Fitó, and Jordi Salas-Salvadó https://pmc.ncbi.nlm.nih.gov/articles/PMC5572601/

Websites:

https://www.healthline.com/health/polyphenols-foods#risks-and-complications

https://health.clevelandclinic.org/polyphenols

https://zoe.com/learn/foods-high-in-polyphenols

www.ingramcontent.com/pod-product-compliance
Lightning Source LLC
Chambersburg PA
CBHW072145090426
42739CB00013B/3285